There Must be More

KELLIE FINLAYSON
with ALLEY PASCOE

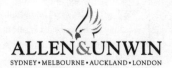

The content presented in this book is meant for inspiration and informational purposes only. The purchaser of this book understands that the author is not a medical professional, and the information contained within this book is not intended to replace medical advice or to be relied upon to treat, cure or prevent any disease, illness or medical condition. It is understood that you will seek full medical clearance by a licensed physician before making any changes mentioned in this book. The author and publisher claim no responsibility to any person or entity for any liability, loss or damage caused or alleged to be caused directly or indirectly as a result of the use, application or interpretation of the material in this book.

First published in 2025

Copyright © Kellie Finlayson, 2025

All rights reserved. No part of this book may be reproduced or transmitted in any form or by any means, electronic or mechanical, including photocopying, recording or by any information storage and retrieval system, without prior permission in writing from the publisher. The Australian *Copyright Act 1968* (the Act) allows a maximum of one chapter or 10 per cent of this book, whichever is the greater, to be photocopied by any educational institution for its educational purposes provided that the educational institution (or body that administers it) has given a remuneration notice to the Copyright Agency (Australia) under the Act.

Allen & Unwin
Cammeraygal Country
83 Alexander Street
Crows Nest NSW 2065
Australia
Phone: (61 2) 8425 0100
Email: info@allenandunwin.com
Web: www.allenandunwin.com

Allen & Unwin acknowledges the Traditional Owners of the Country on which we live and work. We pay our respects to all Aboriginal and Torres Strait Islander Elders, past and present.

 A catalogue record for this book is available from the National Library of Australia

ISBN 978 1 76147 204 6

Set in 12.75/19.5 pt Minion Pro by Midland Typesetters, Australia
Printed and bound in Australia by the Opus Group

10 9 8 7 6 5 4 3 2 1

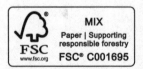 The paper in this book is FSC® certified. FSC® promotes environmentally responsible, socially beneficial and economically viable management of the world's forests.

Contents

Prologue		ix
1	A portaloo joke saved my life	1
2	Two lines and a smiley face	15
3	Hindsight	27
4	Dot, dot, dot	41
5	Baby's first Christmas	55
6	The long, dark night	67
7	Silence as an act of survival	83
8	Three words	107
9	The true cost	127
10	Voice of reason	143
11	Not applicable	161
12	Disguised blessings	179
13	One foot in front of the other	197
14	A non-ideal world	213
15	Remember me	229
Acknowledgements		243
Kellie Finlayson and Jodi Lee Bowel Cancer Foundation		247

*To my younger self, the newly diagnosed, in-shock
and shit-scared me. You've got this. Hold on.
You're stronger than you know.*

*To the reader holding this book:
Have you ever felt your life stop mid-sentence?
Like you're mid-breath, mid-thought, mid-dream,
and then—BAM—it's all gone?
That was me.
I was 25 and running full speed
when the word 'cancer' hit me so hard
I'm still recovering from the whiplash.
Life has a funny way of changing, bending, sometimes breaking.
And I've learned that you either sit there staring at the pieces
or you figure out how to make something new.
I hope my story inspires you.
Create something new.*

Prologue

I've always held a vision for what I wanted my wedding day to be. I pictured the ceremony happening in my home town of Port Lincoln, by the beach overlooking the bay, outside under the sun. I imagined two dresses: one with a big train and veil for the ceremony, and a party dress for dancing at the reception. When Jeremy came into my life, I saw him standing at the end of the aisle.

I knew Jezz was the man I was going to marry. It sounds like a cliché, but it was his eyes that got me: those big blue eyes. I didn't stand a chance. We met at a Justin Bieber concert in Sydney in March 2017, when we were both 21, but we didn't reconnect until after I returned from living overseas a few years later. I had been teaching in Norway, while he'd been making a name for himself in the Australian Football League (AFL), playing for the GWS Giants in Sydney. Then, in

There Must Be More

November 2019, I was in Sydney for the weekend when Jeremy slid into my Instagram DMs. How romantic.

We used to fight all the time about who messaged whom first, but I've got the receipts. It was Jeremy. 'Are you in Sydney?' he asked me. We became inseparable from that moment on.

I will admit, I was the first one to say, 'I love you.' It was Easter 2020. Caramilk had just been reintroduced, changing the chocolate game for those of us too young to have experienced it in the nineties. When Jeremy showed up with a bag of mini Caramilk Easter eggs for me, I gushed, 'I love you.' He said it straight back. 'I've been wanting to say it for ages, but I didn't want to say it first,' he told me.

From the get-go, we were immediately comfortable with each other. I'd be on the toilet while he was in the shower, and vice versa. Nothing was too much. Everything was easy. It was a great feeling. We both wanted the same things out of life: to have a family, a big backyard and a kitchen to cook in together.

We didn't muck around. We moved in together, got a dog and started planning our future. When I fell pregnant in the first year of our relationship, it felt entirely right. We were going to be parents, and we were so excited. Sophia Jai Finlayson was born on 19 August 2021. We were a family. And we moved back to South Australia to be closer to my family.

Prologue

Our daughter was with us in 2022 when Jeremy got down on one knee at Henley Beach, Adelaide, and proposed to me. It was so special to share the moment with her. I was surprised, but I wasn't shocked. I'd sent Jezz a screenshot of the ring I wanted very early on in our relationship; he'd taken my dad out for a beer the night before; and I'd noticed a rather large transaction come out of our joint bank account. Plus, who goes for a 'coffee' at the beach at 3 p.m.? Jezz might not have nailed the art of surprise, but he still blew me away. The ring was beautiful—a simple gold band with an oval diamond set in four delicate claws—and the proposal felt like a natural progression for us. We were going to be together forever. He was mine and I was his. This was it.

I was going to be a bride! On the morning of our wedding on 5 March 2023, I got ready in a hotel room in Adelaide with my bridal party, my parents and Sophia, who was eighteen months old and looked adorable in her little flower-girl dress. We made a bow out of the lace of my veil to put in her hair. She still has it.

When I put my dress on and did the reveal with my mum and dad, the tears began. I arrived in a Mustang at a nondescript cul-de-sac that led down to Tennyson Beach. It was cold and rainy, but that didn't matter. As soon as I saw Jeremy, I felt warm. He was sobbing his eyes out under the arch that was our altar. He wasn't the only one. There wasn't a dry eye on the grass when I walked down the aisle to the Conrad Sewell song 'Remind Me'.

Everyone's eyes were on me, and I didn't know where to look. It was like I could feel the force of everyone's emotions and their love for us. It was overwhelming.

Lucky Sophia was there to bring us all back to reality. In what was meant to be a cute moment in the ceremony, the celebrant asked Soph if Mummy and Daddy could get married. 'No!' she yelled. Righto. Everyone laughed and we carried on (even without her blessing).

Things got all deep and meaningful again when we started our vows. 'Kellie, words cannot explain how truly grateful I am to be marrying you today,' Jeremy said. 'From the moment I met you, I fell in love with you.'

The feeling was mutual. 'Jemison, within the shortest time, I knew it was you . . . It was always you,' I told him.

We promised to love each other endlessly, to be there for each other through the ups and downs, to make each other proud and to be the best parents to our daughter. We promised each other forever.

This should have been the happiest day of our lives, but it wasn't. Underneath the joy was a brutal truth that we couldn't escape, no matter how much we wanted to. As I stood facing Jeremy at the altar, the truth was there with us.

My husband would soon be a widower.

Prologue

Three months earlier

I was breathless. It had started just before Christmas 2022. It felt like I couldn't get enough air into my lungs, like my breaths weren't touching the sides. I tried not to think the worst. I went to the GP and had some tests done. I sucked in more air.

On Boxing Day, it was confirmed.

My bowel cancer had returned.

I had been diagnosed with Stage 4 bowel cancer in November 2021 but, after a year of treatment, I was feeling good. Things were positive. My last round of scans had shown no signs of cancer. Even though my surgeon said he wouldn't use the terms 'remission' or 'cancer-free', he told me he was 'quietly confident'. I held on to that. And when I started struggling to catch my breath, I grasped tighter.

The quiet confidence I had been clinging to was shattered with four words: 'The cancer has spread.'

The oncologist (cancer specialist) recommended palliative care. Jeremy realised—with certainty, for the first time—that he was going to lose me. I found a new oncologist. I was 26. I wasn't going into palliative care; I was going to start another cycle of treatment. It would be a different type of chemo, because I had become allergic to a strand in the treatment I'd had the year before. It was going to be rough.

I was going to lose my hair.

The chemo chair felt chillingly familiar. Sitting in it, I knew we'd have to cancel our wedding. Just a few weeks earlier, we'd sent out save-the-date cards for 13 October 2023. Now we had to message everyone to say the wedding wouldn't be going ahead. They didn't need to save the date anymore.

I didn't want to get married without my hair. In a way, my hair felt like part of my identity. I know that might sound a bit vain, but my attachment to my hair felt more than skin deep. I thought if I lost my hair, everything else would go with it. In my mind, if I looked well, I could be well. If I looked sick, I was going to be sick. I didn't want that. I was sure one of the reasons I'd gotten through my first cycle of chemo was because I didn't look like I was going through chemo. People treated me normally and didn't act like I was dying. If people had wrapped me in cottonwool and looked at me with pity, I would have crumbled.

The thought of losing my hair freaked me out so much because it made losing my life real. I didn't want to be a bald bride—that was true. But the main reason we cancelled the wedding was because we didn't know if I would make it to October. And I didn't want to die with a different last name to my daughter's.

Jeremy and I talked about going to the courthouse to sign a marriage licence and change my last name. We'd come to terms with cancelling our dream wedding, but I hadn't given up hope of getting married. When I mentioned the courthouse idea to my mum, she asked, 'Why don't you just elope?'

Prologue

'If we elope, I want at least our families and my maid of honour there,' I said.

'Well, let's do that, then,' Mum replied.

It was decided. We were going to have a tiny ceremony with our closest family and friends, and we were going to do it in three weeks. I had already started treatment and my hair was beginning to fall out. It wasn't noticeable yet, but I feared it would be soon. Time was ticking.

As soon as the decision was made, we rallied. Our families booked in annual leave to make it. My bridesmaids bought their own dresses. Our photographer offered her services for free, as did our celebrant, and a hotel in the city gifted us three rooms for the bridal party.

I had already cancelled the order for my wedding dress, but when the dress shop, Made with Love Bridal, caught wind of the rushed wedding, it came to save the day. I was quite thin—because I was malnourished—which meant I could fit into a sample size. It also meant that the port I'd just had inserted into my chest for chemo was really sticking out. It was a foreign object in my body, and I wasn't at all used to it yet. I was nervous about getting married with it being so noticeable, but when I put on the dress, all I felt was beautiful. I looked like myself (thanks to some hard work from my hair and make-up artists). I'd always wanted a strapless dress, and the bridal store made me the most stunning gown with a corset that fit me perfectly.

There Must Be More

This wasn't the wedding I had imagined as a little girl. And it wasn't the one I'd planned months earlier. We couldn't make it to Port Lincoln because I needed to stay close to the hospital in Adelaide. We weren't surrounded by our extended family and friends, just 21 of the people closest to us—and some paparazzi in the bushes nearby, taking photos.

I didn't have a second wedding dress for the reception because there wasn't going to be a reception. I was exhausted. We had a nice dinner with everyone and I was ready for bed at 8 p.m. Our first dance as husband and wife was to 'Khe Sanh' by Cold Chisel, in our hotel room, wearing our pyjamas. (That was probably for the best: Jezz is a tragic dancer.)

When the celebrant pronounced us husband and wife and told Jeremy he could kiss the bride, I hesitated. My body was toxic from my chemo treatment, and I didn't want to make Jeremy sick by kissing him and passing on my toxins. We shared our first kiss at the altar, but we staged all the kisses in our photos because I didn't want to risk it. What a wild thought to have on your wedding day: *I can't kiss my husband without making him unwell.*

We didn't consummate our marriage on the night of the wedding, either—despite all the winking and nudging of Jeremy's groomsman! It was a luxury to have a full night's sleep in a hotel bed without Sophia in between us, kicking us all night. It's the little things, you know.

Prologue

We didn't go on a honeymoon after the wedding. Jeremy started the new footy season and I started another round of chemo. At the time, I did have a twinge of sadness. I think it's normal to have expectations for such a big day in your life. I could never have expected I would be terminally ill, at the age of 27, on my wedding day. No one imagines walking down the aisle with a chemo port in their chest.

Now, looking back, I know our wedding played out the way it was meant to. We were all just stoked that it was happening at all. Everyone at the wedding knew I was unwell, of course, but no one spoke about it. There was an elephant in the room, but we didn't let it ruin the day. We couldn't change reality, but we could have a little break from it. Just for one day.

I was so grateful to everyone who made our wedding day what it was. So many people went above and beyond for us. I had been happy to settle for a simple wedding band, because the one I had always wanted was $10,000 and we couldn't justify that with the cost of my health care. A wedding band wasn't a priority. When Jeremy's teammate at Port Adelaide, Travis Boak, found out about my dream ring, he made it his priority to make it happen for me. He went to all the boys at the club and got them to chuck in some money. The rushed wedding was still a secret, so Travis said, 'Look, Kellie and Jeremy need help with something. Do you want to put in for it?' Not one person questioned it. They put their hands in their pockets. That's how the boys at Port Adelaide ended up paying for my wedding band. Say no more. To this day, Trav—the humble bloke he is—doesn't realise how much of an impact he had on our wedding day.

The love we felt for each other on and around our wedding day was something else. We might not have had a big party reception or a proper first dance, but we had each other.

Two months earlier, I'd been told to go home and get comfortable. And yet, I was still standing. Not just standing, but walking down the aisle to the love of my life. I'll never forget that moment.

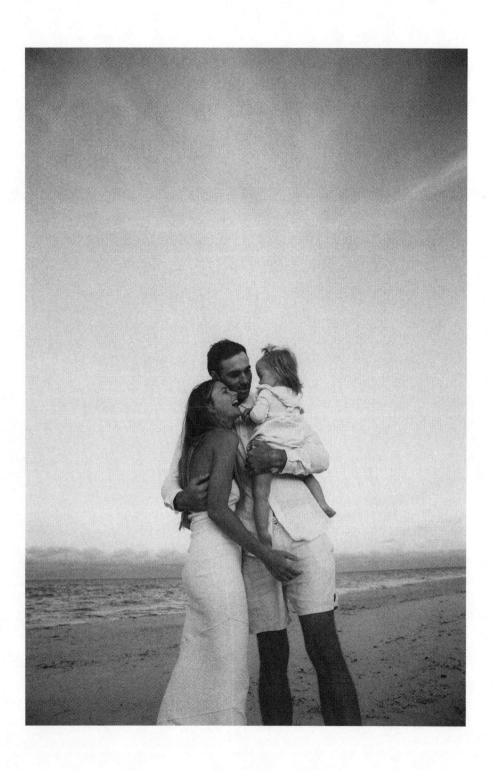

1
A portaloo joke saved my life

'Please pull over, Jezz,' I begged. 'I'm going to shit myself.'

There are five petrol stations on the 40-minute drive from Adelaide to the lolly shop in Hahndorf, in the Adelaide Hills. I know because we stopped at all of them, me urgently needing to go to the bathroom.

At the first petrol station, I grabbed a bottle of water, an apple, and a doughnut with sprinkles in a plastic wrapper. And I made sure I went to the toilet. It was early on a Sunday morning, and I'd just breastfed Sophia, who was almost three months old, in the hope that she'd sleep in the car on the drive.

'Alright, are you good to go?' Jeremy asked me.

'Yep, I think so,' I said, running through the road-trip checklist: fuel, snacks, toilet. Coffee. We needed coffee!

It was in the queue at the drive-through coffee place that I realised I needed to go to the bathroom again. Urgently.

I thought I'd finished my business at the first stop, but I obviously had more to do. I made Jeremy drive around to the next window so I could ask to use the bathroom inside.

'It's a drive-through, babe. They won't have a toilet here,' said Jezz, shaking his head ever so slightly as I leaned over him to speak to the woman in the window.

'We don't normally let customers use the staff bathroom,' the cashier said hesitantly.

'Please, I really need to go. I've just had a baby.' I nodded to Sophia in her car seat in the back. The cashier took pity on me and my pelvic floor, and let me in for a wee. I didn't need a wee, though; I desperately needed to do a poo. But when I sat on the toilet, nothing came out. Not even a fart. I had the urge to go, but I couldn't. I sat there for a few more minutes before giving up and going back to the car.

'Did you go?' Jeremy asked me as I jumped in the passenger seat.

'Yep,' I lied, not wanting him to think we'd stopped for no reason.

By the third bathroom stop on our drive to the countryside, Jeremy was understandably getting annoyed. I'd just been to the bathroom twice in fifteen minutes, and I needed to go again.

'Fuck's sake,' Jezz said, pulling into another petrol station. 'We need to hire a portaloo! We're pulling over every fifty metres, and it's not even because of the baby.'

I didn't clap back at him because I was busy clenching my bum and rushing inside. I pushed open the cubicle door, shimmied down my pants and sat on the toilet seat. There was a tiny splash. All that for *that*.

'That's it, we're getting a portaloo.' Jezz repeated his joke when I got back to the car.

'It's not funny! Don't joke about it. There's clearly something wrong. I'm postpartum. Something's going on.'

'Yeah, I get that. You need to see a doctor Kell,' Jeremy insisted. 'You need to do something about it. It's not just affecting your life, it's affecting *our* life.'

'Oh yeah, because pulling over every now and then is so hard,' I said defensively.

But Jeremy was right and I knew it. There was something wrong, and I needed to do something about it. I picked up my phone and googled 'bulk-billing doctors near me'. I moved the map to our suburb in Adelaide, found a GP clinic and booked the next available appointment. On the online form, I explained that I was having bowel issues and wanted to see a doctor. The appointment was scheduled for three days later. It took less than five minutes to set up, and when we eventually pulled up in Hahndorf after our highway servo tour I thought nothing more of it.

At the lolly shop, I bought all my favourites: white chocolate–coated raspberry liquorice, FruChocs and white chocolate freckles. Jeremy got a giant chocolate frog.

We were like two kids in a candy store (because we were)—three, if you included the actual child, Sophia, whom we'd used as an excuse to stop into my favourite lolly shop in the countryside. We were loving being new parents and were still bouncing around in the baby bubble, hence the spontaneous drive. But that 2021 road trip to the Hahndorf lolly shop would set off a chain of events that would blow up my entire life.

For so long, all I had wanted was to get out and see the world. In my childhood bedroom in Port Lincoln—on the Eyre Peninsula, a seven-hour drive from Adelaide, population 14,000—I'd so often thought to myself, *There must be more out there.* I'd worked so hard to make it out, yet now I was back in my home state of South Australia after years abroad and interstate. And I thank the universe every day that I was home.

There was nowhere else I could have faced what was to come.

~

Port Lincoln is the kind of place where everyone knows everyone and their cousin. There are two pubs—one at each end of town—a sports field in the middle and a wharf out over the water. Growing up, we lived on the outskirts of town: me, my mum, Jane, my dad, Jeff, and my younger brother, Jake. The three Js and me.

We lived in a typical three-bedroom, one-bathroom house with a big backyard. It was an ordinary house and an ordinary childhood. Mum was an accountant and Dad was a mechanic and diesel tuner. Interestingly, Dad was better at helping me with my maths homework than Mum. Even more interestingly, both of my parents were adopted. Mum was born in Adelaide and adopted by Norwegian parents who lived in Port Lincoln. Dad was born in Whyalla, three hours northeast, and ended up in Port Lincoln, too. My parents met in high school; they got married on Mum's nineteenth birthday, bought a house together and had me five years later.

The story goes that, when Mum's waters broke, she didn't go to the hospital. She went to the supermarket. She did a grocery shop for my dad because he would've starved on his own. Theirs was a traditional marriage. Mum did the cleaning, cooking and shopping—even when she was in labour. After grabbing the groceries, Mum went home, had a bath and waited for Dad to finish work at 5 p.m. They went to the hospital together and I was born an hour later.

I was a boy until I was born. Mum and Dad didn't ask to find out my sex, but at a scan, they mistook a foot for a penis and guessed I was a boy.

'That's a girl,' Dad said when I came out. Surprise!

Mum and Dad have lived in the same house my whole life. I grew up knowing all our neighbours and having a best friend who lived just down the street and around the corner. An Italian family with two girls around my age lived across the road from us, and I would go to church with them every Sunday because I knew there'd be lunch afterwards and the food was the best thing ever. It was such a good upbringing.

Fun fact: when I was one, my grandpa on my mum's side won the lottery. Grandpa paid off Mum and Dad's mortgage with some of his winnings. It wasn't a huge amount of money—back then, people could actually afford to buy a house—but it was a big help for Mum and Dad. In return, they gave Grandpa a grandson. That's how Jake came along.

My brother's bedroom was opposite mine, and I used to get the belt from my dressing gown and tie his doorknob to mine so he'd be stuck in his room. The harder he pulled, the tighter the knots would get. It was the only way I could get away from him. My brother was hard work. He was diagnosed with ADHD when getting a diagnosis was much more difficult and less common than it is today. My parents had their hands full with Jake, so I just kind of did my own thing. I was always independent and confident. I don't know if I was born that way or if I became that way because I had to.

I was lucky. I was academic and athletic. My teachers liked me because I was a good student, but I talked a lot and was secretly cheeky. I remember swapping my mouse cord with the computer opposite me in the computer lab—remember those?—so the other kid's mouse would be useless. He'd get frustrated and I'd step in to fix the issue.

'Do you want me to help him, Miss?' I'd offer.

I was a good kid and I didn't get into any major trouble, unlike my brother. I can imagine it would have been pretty hard for Jake walking in his older sister's shadow. He wasn't as sporty or as studious; Mum used to bribe him with $50 for every A he could get on his report card. Meanwhile, mine was full of As, but I didn't get a cash incentive. Ripped off, hey.

At Jake's first football game when he was seven or eight, he refused to play, so I ended up taking to the field for him. Growing up in South Australia, AFL was huge. Whenever an AFL player came to Port Lincoln, it was like a celebrity was in town. They were worshipped like gods. My parents are Adelaide Crows supporters, but I went for Collingwood—the black-and-white Magpies—because my junior netball team had a black-and-white uniform. It made sense to me to colour coordinate my loyalty.

I played every sport under the sun. I started dancing when I was two and competing at age four. I also played basketball, netball, tennis and indoor soccer. I loved soccer because I got to play against my brother. I always beat him, which was amazing. When I was eight, I started to learn how to sail. They held lessons and races in the bay at Port Lincoln. I did it for years and got quite good. Okay, I probably wasn't that good; there were only like twenty other boats competing, and I didn't win very often. Still, that didn't stop me from dreaming about going to the Olympics, like kids do. After years of asking, my mum finally bought me my own holdy—a small sailing boat. A week later, a shark was found in the bay. Mum sold the holdy. My sailing—and Olympic—dreams were over.

Not to worry: there were so many other sports to keep me occupied. I spent a lot of time going away with my different teams. We did trips across South Australia to Whyalla, Port Augusta, Port Pirie and Adelaide to compete at state and national levels. Whether I was conscious of it or not, I somehow chose to compete in all the sports that involved travelling for comps. Now I see it was my way of getting out. I knew there was more to the world than the limits of Port Lincoln, and I wanted to experience it.

It was only after spending more time in Adelaide—or 'the big smoke' as we called it—and making new friends outside of my home town that I realised how toxic the friendship circles were back home. Everyone knew absolutely everything about everyone in Lincoln. There was no privacy. Make a mistake, and you'd be reminded of it. I hated it.

The limits of Port Lincoln were well defined, and I felt them closing in on me. I was far too adventurous to be the small-town girl. Sure, it is a beautiful town to bring up a family or retire; but I didn't feel like it was a place where I could chase my dreams, challenge myself or push boundaries.

Small towns move at their own pace: slow. I moved at a different speed: quick.

~

It all happened so fast. After I booked my GP appointment during our trip to the Hahndorf lolly shop, someone at the clinic rang me and said they'd brought the appointment forward. I was due to take baby Sophia to her twelve-week check-up, so they organised to do that at the same time as seeing me. I walked into the clinic expecting to weigh my baby, talk some shit (literally) and leave with a jar for a stool sample.

I was relieved to find I'd been booked in to see a female doctor, probably because I was postpartum.

'Okay, tell me. What's going on?' the doctor asked me when I sat down with Sophia in my arms.

'It's actually my bowels,' I revealed.

We ran through the list of usual suspects.

'I'm not gluten or lactose intolerant, so I thought that I might have IBS? Just because of the inflammation and the blood in my stool.'

The doctor's face changed.

'You've had what in your stool?' she asked.

'Blood,' I repeated. 'Not regularly, just a once-off every now and then.'

'When was the first time you had it?'

'At the start of 2020.'

'So, nearly two years ago?' The doctor was clearly not impressed. For the first time, I got a sense that things might be more serious than I thought. The doctor wrote me a referral for a specialist, and I was booked in for an appointment with them in a couple of weeks.

The next day the phone rang. 'I've got an opening this afternoon at 4 p.m.,' the specialist told me. 'Can you make it?'

I jumped at the early appointment, figuring that the GP I'd seen had put in a good word for me. *It pays to know people in high places*, I thought to myself. When I met the specialist, he organised for me to have a colonoscopy the next day. Again, I thought I'd lucked out. I started the bowel prep—taking laxatives to clear the bowels and electrolytes to prevent dehydration—right away.

The timing wasn't ideal. Jeremy was working—doing a promo event at Adelaide Oval—so I was bowel prepping and parenting on my own. I couldn't breastfeed Sophia because I was taking laxatives, so I was giving her formula for the first time. The doctor had warned me: once you drink the laxatives, you'll be glued to the toilet. After I downed the first litre, nothing happened. I should've known then. But I didn't, so I drank another litre. I was so full that the liquid started coming back up. I spewed the bowel prep up, not realising that it was because it couldn't get out the other end. Something was in the way.

A portaloo joke saved my life

I was in the foetal position in the shower, spewing and doing tiny squirts of poo. Baby Sophia fell asleep on the bath mat outside the shower. I felt like the worst mother. 'I'm so sorry, baby,' I whispered to my sleeping daughter.

'Please come home,' I begged Jeremy, after finally relenting and calling him. When he did, Sophia was still asleep on the bathroom floor, and I was in tears because I couldn't keep the second litre of laxatives down. I called the specialist's office to tell them, and they told me not to worry, that the first litre usually did the trick. I didn't know how to explain that next to nothing had come out of my bowels. And I didn't want to, in case they made me go through the entire process again.

The next afternoon, my colonoscopy was delayed by three hours. I was starving because I hadn't eaten and had spewed everything inside me out. I felt empty in every sense. When the procedure finally happened, it lasted ten seconds. I woke up from the anaesthetic, saw the clock and looked at the nurses. 'That didn't take long,' I said to them.

'No, dear, it doesn't take long,' they said. It was reassuring.

It shouldn't have been. The reason it was so quick was because the doctor couldn't physically perform the colonoscopy. My tumour was so big, it was blocking the way.

I was a bit out of it after the anaesthesia, but I remember thinking how lovely everyone was being to me. The nurses were so kind and helpful. When I got dressed and walked to the reception area, Jeremy was sitting with Sophia, waiting for me. I wasn't expecting them to be there; the hospital's Covid restrictions were tight. I assumed they made an exception for us because I was the last patient of the day and we had a little baby. *That's so sweet of them*, I thought to myself, groggily.

We were ushered into the gastroenterologist's office. The doctor was looking at a piece of paper. He turned it around to show us. 'This is what bowel cancer looks like,' he said.

He was holding a photo of my bowel.

I went completely blank. I didn't understand. 'What do you mean?' I asked.

Jeremy had his own questions. 'What the fuck is happening?' he said, as he passed Sophia to a nurse to hold. He was in shock.

'You have bowel cancer. I'm sorry, I don't know what else to say,' the doctor replied.

I have bowel cancer.

'I've already messaged a surgeon at a private hospital,' the doctor continued. 'He will see you tomorrow at four-fifteen p.m.'

I need surgery.

'We'll talk again. You need some time to process this,' the doctor added.

Fuck.

I got up and left the room. I still had a cannula in my arm. When the nurse tried to tell me she had to take it out before I left, I kept walking. 'Please, don't,' I said.

I was rattled. And I was angry. I didn't want to be touched. I wanted to go home. I was hungry. I wanted to get something to eat. More than anything, I wanted to rewind the last few hours and go back to before. Before I had cancer. Before I needed surgery. *Before.*

'I'm just really not in the mood to be here,' I told the nurse, who was trying to reason with me about the cannula. I was being such a brat, but I wasn't functioning normally. After some wrangling, they finally got the cannula out of me and I was free to leave the hospital. I walked to our car and buckled Sophia into her car seat in a daze. I sat next to her in the back seat and held her hand. She was so tiny. Her little fingers curled around my thumb.

Jeremy did the only thing he could think of. He called my mum. 'I don't know how to tell you this, but Kellie has cancer,' he said.

I heard the words he said, but I didn't understand them. In the background of the call, I was howling with tears. The noises I was making were primal; animalistic. And terrifying. I sobbed until the tears stopped coming, until I realised crying wasn't going to solve anything, and something else took over. Shock. A complete overwhelm. Nothing made sense, no emotion felt like the right one.

Jeremy doesn't remember the drive home from the hospital. He was operating on autopilot. He must have called my two good friends, because they were there when we got home. They offered to help put Sophia to bed, and I snapped.

'No. She's my baby, I'll put her to bed,' I said. 'I got a diagnosis, I'm not fucking dead.'

I was in shock. And denial. I tried to make sense of the senseless.

I have bowel cancer.

I need surgery.

Fuck.

2
Two lines and a smiley face

There's nothing sexy about shit. Unless you're a plumber on a job site or a nurse on duty, talking about excrement is pretty taboo in everyday life. It's uncomfortable, unpleasant and embarrassing. So, for many years, I suffered in silence.

I've had issues with my stomach since 2017, when I was 21. My bowel movements have been wildly irregular; sometimes I wouldn't shit for days, and other times I couldn't stop going. I figured I had IBS or coeliac disease. Having a gluten intolerance was all the rage at the time—everyone was going gluten free. I almost rolled my eyes thinking I'd be joining the club. I was more annoyed than concerned about my tummy. It was frustrating being so infrequent, but I didn't think it was anything serious, so I didn't treat it as such.

At the start of 2020, I was living in a townhouse in Melbourne with a couple of girlfriends and working as a relief teacher at Loreto girls' school. I'd started seeing Jeremy; we were doing the long-distance thing, as he was playing for the Giants in Sydney. It was while I was in Melbourne that I went to see a naturopath. I wanted to get to the bottom of what was going on with me—and my bottom. The girlfriends I was living with had noticed how much I was going to the bathroom and asked me if I was okay. I wasn't. At the naturopath, I did an allergy test, and it came back clean; I wasn't intolerant to anything. I could cross ~~coeliac disease~~ off my list. The naturopath gave me a gut reset supplement cleanse, in case I had a parasite. I didn't have a ~~parasite~~.

Then I found blood in my poo.

I went to the GP and they told me I was probably wiping too hard or going too frequently, which I was, so that made sense. I did a stool sample anyway and dropped it off the next day. There was mucus in the stool, so they sent it away for testing. I wasn't just ~~wiping too hard~~. There was a discrepancy in the sample, so they booked me in for a colonoscopy for 23 March 2020.

Then the world shut down.

The Friday before my appointment, I was walking along St Kilda esplanade with a friend, coffee in hand, when my phone rang. It was the day surgery where my colonoscopy was scheduled. The person on the other end of the line explained that all elective procedures had been cancelled because of the new Covid-19 restrictions, so my colonoscopy was off.

In the moment, I was relieved because I didn't need to do the bowel prep.

Because my colonoscopy was considered 'elective surgery', I once again figured it wasn't that serious. If it was important, they wouldn't have cancelled the procedure.

I mentally removed 'colonoscopy' from my to-do list and replaced it with 'get through the pandemic'. It was an almighty task. Schools went online, businesses closed their doors, Melbourne locked down and the AFL season came to a halt. Jeremy was home alone in Sydney; his games had been cancelled indefinitely. That's when I decided to make the move north. We'd been exclusively dating for five months when I moved in with him. It was the easiest decision I've ever made.

That was June. Come the last week of July, we were on the move again. The AFL had created a quarantine hub on the Gold Coast where players, their families and team staff were sent to live and train. As if moving in together wasn't enough, we were forced into the close confines of a Covid bubble. I felt lucky to be there, though. The rules were that only partners who lived or had kids together could join the hub, so I was grateful I'd moved in with Jeremy the month before. I felt for some of the other partners—especially those with little kids—who had to choose between uprooting their entire lives to move to Queensland or staying put and being separated from their partner for an undisclosed period of time. I was a free agent in many ways; my relief teaching contract at Loreto had finished so I wasn't tied down to a job or city.

Living in the hub didn't feel like real life. It was almost like being on school camp—or a *Love Island*–esque reality TV show, minus the partner swapping and over-produced drama. The players and partners in the hub became a tight unit. We didn't see people outside the hub. We were allowed to go for walks outside and grab takeaway coffees, but we couldn't go to restaurants or shopping centres.

Jeremy's parents—Gordon and Carol—had moved to Queensland, but we didn't get to see much of them because of the tight restrictions. Jezz grew up in Culcairn, in the Murray region of New South Wales, close to the Victorian border. He is a Yorta Yorta man, and he grew up with his two brothers and a sister. His dad worked at the Kapooka army base and his mum worked at the local butcher's. Jezz is the definition of a small-town boy done good. When he moved to Sydney at age sixteen to chase his footy dreams, he went from living in a town of 950 people to going to a school with 1200 kids. Justin Bieber might have brought us together, but we definitely bonded over our small-town upbringings.

In the hub, I spent a lot of time with the other partners and their little ones. There wasn't any on-the-ground support from friends or relatives, so I was happy to lend a helping hand. The kids followed me around and I became like a mama hen to them. They started calling me Kell-a-melon, and the nickname stuck. Their mums started jokingly asking me when I was going to have one of my own.

I tried to treat the hub like a holiday, which was pretty easy when I was sitting at the pool in the Queensland sun most days.

We were back in Sydney in January 2021, during the off season, when my phone rang. The hospital in Melbourne was ringing to reschedule my colonoscopy. It was ten months after the procedure had been cancelled, and I was unable to rebook it. Not because I'd moved states—because I was pregnant!

~

It was two days before Christmas. We were in Queensland, where Jeremy's parents lived, and where my family had travelled to from Port Lincoln to spend the holidays with us. My boobs were really sore. Putting a bikini top on was excruciating. I'd never felt anything like it. I was due for my period, so I chalked it up to that at first. On 23 December 2020, I was in a grocery store packed with mask-clad pre-Christmas shoppers. My boobs were still aching—and huge!—so I grabbed a pregnancy test. I doubted I was pregnant, but I figured I might as well do the test.

I was in a shopping-centre toilet cubicle when I found out. It was a happy surprise. When I saw the two lines appear on the stick, I wasn't scared. I was only excited. Jeremy and

I hadn't been trying to have a baby, but we weren't *not* trying. We both wanted kids and knew they were in our future. We were 25 (me) and 24 (him), and we had our shit together. That might seem young to some people, but we knew what we were capable of and what we wanted in life. We wanted to have a family together, and we were going to.

I'd only purchased one pregnancy test, the cheapest I could find, so I went back to the grocery store to get one of the fancy ones that tells you how many weeks you are. Somehow, I squeezed out some more wee in the toilet cubicle, but only a smiley face appeared. Fuck, I'd gotten the wrong test. Back to the grocery store I went, carrying eight shopping bags, to buy a third pregnancy test. I don't know what the cashier must have thought.

Third time lucky, the test revealed that I was three-plus weeks pregnant. The first person I called was Jeremy's best friend, Zac (Williams, who played for the Giants with Jezz). He was stressed out Christmas shopping for his new girlfriend, Rachel.

'Mmm, yeah, do you think I should get a pair of baby socks or a little onesie for Jeremy?' I asked him.

'What do you mean?' he replied.

I spelled it out. 'Zac, I'm pregnant.'

'Oh my god!' He burst into tears.

'I need your help. How do I tell Jezz?'

'Don't tell him now,' he suggested. 'Wait until Christmas.'

Yeah, right. That was never going to happen. I was bursting to tell Jeremy. I made Zac promise to act surprised and not tell Jezz he knew before him, and I threw a plan together. Jeremy's mum had given me his childhood Santa sack from when he was a kid because it was our first Christmas together, and I decided to put the pregnancy test and some baby gear in there. I put the Santa sack in his bedside table, and when Jezz got home I asked him to grab a hairbrush out of the bedside table for me. He did as he was told and moved the Santa sack out of the way to look for the hairbrush.

'It's not even in here,' Jeremy said.

'Oh, it might be in your Santa sack,' I prompted.

'Why would it be in my Santa sack?' he didn't bite.

I gave up. I'd wanted to do a cute surprise like the ones you see on Instagram, but I'd messed it up.

'I'm pregnant! Look in your Santa sack. I've ruined the surprise,' I said.

'So there's no hairbrush?' Jeremy replied, before it sunk in. 'Oh, Kell! Have you told your mum?'

He was so excited. I wanted to celebrate the moment together before telling anyone, but that lasted an hour before I couldn't wait any longer. We planned how to tell our parents. We got a couple of babies' dummies on the way to my parents' holiday rental, and wrapped them up. As we handed over the present I asked my brother to film the moment.

'Oh my god, are you sending them on a holiday?' he asked.

'It's something they've always wanted . . .' I hinted.

When Mum opened the present, she clicked straight away and started tearing up immediately. Dad took a minute. 'Are these for the dog?' he asked, knowing that we treated our dog, Henley, like a little baby.

The tears in Mum's eyes must have tipped Dad off. They were both over the moon for us. It was such a special moment.

I kept it real. 'Can we have the dummies back, though? They're expensive.'

After telling our families, the next people I told were the girls from the hub, the ones who kept asking me when I was going to have a baby of my own. They were all stoked for us, and for their kids who were going to have a new little friend. It wasn't until after Sophia was born that I told Jeremy the very first person who knew about the baby was his best mate, Zac.

To celebrate the happy news, my mum, ever the accountant, bought me private health insurance. It was a congratulatory gift—a very practical one at that—and I appreciated it.

No one could have known just how important that gift was going to be.

We found out we were having a girl. I knew our daughter was going to have Jeremy wrapped around her finger. I couldn't wait.

I had a textbook, stock-standard pregnancy, except for one thing: I developed varicose veins down the insides of my legs. They were all over my vulva, too, and they were incredibly painful. I couldn't sit down half the time. It was brutal. I'd never heard of anyone experiencing that kind of pressure on their blood vessels, but I chalked it up to pregnancy.

Towards the end of my pregnancy, I had a lot of abdominal pain, and I was worried about the baby's positioning. I went for several scans to try to determine what was causing the pain. They all came back clear. There was nothing wrong with me or the baby, according to the scans.

My waters broke at 37 weeks. It was only my hind waters, though, and the baby's head plugged the flow. There was no meconium in the fluid, so I was given an antibiotic and the doctors told me to sit tight. I crossed my legs and tried to relax. At the time we were staying in an Airbnb overlooking a marina on the Gold Coast that we'd booked for six weeks. We'd always spoken about living in a house on the water, so we got a kick out of being there. It was beautiful.

Jeremy eventually decided to hang up his boots for the season. There were only a few rounds left in it, and if he kept playing, he would've had to travel to Western Australia. The border could close any day, and he didn't want to risk being stuck on the other side of the country, away from me and our soon-to-be-born child. He chose to stay.

I knew it was a difficult call for Jeremy to make. It was even harder when GWS made the semifinals and Jezz wasn't able to take the field alongside his teammates. He was devastated, obviously. We watched the game on TV at our Airbnb in Queensland and cheered them on from afar. I don't know if it was more painful or less for Jeremy when they lost.

At 39 weeks, my waters broke for a second time. I left puddles with every step I took. When I admitted myself to hospital, though, I was only three centimetres dilated. I wasn't in any pain; my contractions weren't hurting at all. The midwife suggested that I go home, have a warm shower and wait it out there. It was 11 p.m. I thought I'd go home and get some sleep, but then remembered lying down can slow labour. So, I kept standing.

I stood under the shower until it ran out of hot water. Come morning, I ate breakfast and figured I'd killed enough time. We went back to the hospital at 7 a.m. and were put into the most beautiful room with Aboriginal paintings on the walls. I was given Pitocin (a synthetic version of oxytocin) to speed up my contractions. It worked—a little too well. I went from having no pain to the worst pain I've ever felt. For four hours straight, I had nonstop contractions. I tried sitting on an exercise ball under the shower, but it didn't help. Jeremy had to hold me up because I kept falling backwards.

Eventually I was given an epidural, which worked on one side of my body. I could lie on my numb left side and bear the pain. Day turned to night, turned to morning. The labour went on and on. The baby wasn't budging. At one point, a midwife pulled a pair of scissors out.

'Get those away from me!' I said. I didn't want to be cut.

At 3 a.m., Jezz told me he was going to shut his eyes for 30 minutes. Ten minutes later, our baby was born.

Sophia was everything we'd ever dreamed of. Ten little fingers and ten little toes; our baby girl. Holding her in my arms felt surreal.

People make out that birth is a magical experience—and it is—but it's also pretty gruesome. I was spewing so much during the final stages of labour I basically vomited Sophia out. Once she was born, my placenta wouldn't birth, so the midwife told me I'd have to go in for surgery.

'Nup, I just avoided surgery. Can't you get it out here?'

'Okay, but it's messy . . .' she warned me.

'I just had a baby,' I said. *How bad could it be?* I thought.

I nearly ate my words when the midwife flicked a pair of gloves on, like a scene in a horror film. I was half-numb thanks to the epidural, so Jeremy had to tell me what was going on down there. He slapped his elbow to indicate the midwife was elbow-deep inside me, digging to retrieve my placenta. When it came out, the placenta was lacerated, like a steak chopped up. It wasn't pretty.

Later, I asked Jeremy if I shit myself during the birth.

'So much!' he exclaimed.

I'd never given birth before, so I didn't know what to expect. I thought the things I went through—the varicose veins, abdominal pain and lacerated placenta—were normal parts of growing and birthing a child. They weren't. They were signs. There was a tumour inside me and my baby had been pushing down on it, which led to the pressure and the pain and the sliced placenta.

I had so many scans, ultrasounds and appointments during my pregnancy. Looking back, I have wondered, *How the fuck didn't they see the enormous tumour right there?* I talked to a sonographer, and they explained that when someone is doing a scan, they're just looking at the targeted area—which in this case was my uterus and baby.

If only they had looked at my bowel.

3
Hindsight

I lied to get out of the hospital. When Sophia was born, she was in the neonatal intensive care unit (NICU) because of the trauma of her birth. I was allocated a separate room in the maternity ward, but I slept on the couch in the NICU beside Soph instead. I was desperate to get out of the hospital, and to take my baby with me. When the nurse was doing her discharge checks with me, she asked if I'd had a bowel movement since giving birth. 'Yes,' I lied.

We left the hospital for our temporary home, the Airbnb on the Gold Coast marina, where my mum was waiting for us having flown up from South Australia to meet her first grandchild. It was August and the Queensland sun welcomed us home.

Then, ten days after giving birth, I was in total agony. I told Mum how sick I was.

'Just go to the toilet,' she advised. 'Take a laxative if you need.'

'Mum, I'm scared.' I admitted I hadn't gone to the toilet since before Sophia was born.

I had a ten-day-old baby and I was in so much pain, I couldn't feed her. It was dire. I took three different types of laxatives, drank four litres of water, had two enemas and a suppository. I tried desperately to get my bowels to move. I ended up lying on the shower floor in the foetal position, pushing watery, pencil-thin poo out of myself. It was the most disturbing experience of my life—and I'd just given birth! I'm so glad Mum was there to help me, because Jeremy would have been beside himself if he had to see me like that.

Once again, I chalked my severe constipation up to pregnancy, birth and the epidural. I figured everything down there was swollen and stressed, and that what I was going through was normal. Everyone knows the first poo after having a baby is brutal. Mine was no exception.

After that dreadful day on the shower floor, my bowels woke up a little. But I still wasn't regular. When I did finally go, I kept feeling like I had to *keep* going. I can't explain the urgency. I was sure I was going to shit myself, but when I got to the nearest toilet, most of the time nothing came out. It felt like there was a poo constantly waiting to escape.

I called Jeremy's team doctor and asked him if I might have haemorrhoids. He told me it was definitely a possibility after birth, and if I had a feel around my anus I'd be able to tell if there were haemorrhoids. I did feel something. I didn't know then it wasn't haemorrhoids.

My body might have been in the wars, but I was loving being a mum. I know I'm entirely biased, but Sophia was the most gorgeous baby. She had Jeremy's bright blue eyes and a perfect little button nose. I felt so lucky to be her mum, and to get to watch Jeremy be her dad.

We were a family, and we wanted to be surrounded by family. We needed support. Jeremy still had two years on his contract with the Giants in Sydney, but we didn't have anyone close to us there. I was afraid of being isolated in a city with a newborn baby and without any family nearby. We went to the team manager and explained our concerns. We wanted to move closer to my family, and hoped we could discuss the potential of a trade. The team understood, and were happy for Jeremy to explore his options, but they couldn't make any promises until the trade period began.

When Sophia was three weeks old, we left Queensland for South Australia. We were going down to be with my family, and also so Jeremy could meet with the team at Port Adelaide Football Club. It was some secret-squirrel stuff. Jezz had to enter the meeting through a back door because he couldn't risk being seen and having it leaked to the media.

Of course, it was leaked anyway. It was all over the news that Jeremy was in Adelaide. We were holed up in an Adelaide hotel with our newborn baby while Jeremy was having trade meetings over Zoom. He had some serious interest from the Hawthorn team in Melbourne. Jezz knew the coach there and got on really well with him. We had friends in Melbourne, but the whole point of the trade was to move closer to family.

At the Port Adelaide grounds, Jeremy had a medical and did a round of fitness tests with their team doctor and another impartial doctor. From there, we travelled to Port Lincoln to stay with my parents, and had three weeks together, just living. It was amazing. The weather turned it up for us and we spent our days at the beach, and whale-watching at the lookout with our little baby. Sophia was in a really good routine, feeding every three hours during the day and having five-hour sleeps overnight. We would put her down at 7 p.m. and do a dream feed at 9 p.m. as I was going to bed, and she would sleep until 3 a.m., followed by another three or four hours after another feed. If I wanted a full sleep, Mum would do the 3 a.m. feed with a bottle of pumped breastmilk. Sophia was such a good baby, and those few weeks at home were such a special time.

A Stan series—*Show Me the Money*—was being filmed about the AFL trade period, so a TV crew flew into Port Lincoln to capture footage of Jeremy and our family. I was having a morning coffee with a girlfriend who'd also just had a baby when the cameras started rolling. I didn't even have my breast pads on! I was worried about having leaking boobs and a screaming baby in every shot. They filmed us for an entire day and it was wild. We'd never experienced anything like it. In Sydney, there was no noise around the AFL. Players and their families could do anything without being noticed. When we lived there, we could go to a cafe and not one person would recognise Jeremy. The only time I saw someone approach him, they asked vaguely if he was an athlete. 'Nah, mate, I'm a plumber,' he replied.

It was a different story in Port Lincoln—the land of AFL. Everyone knew Jezz was a footy player, so he got plenty of looks and g'days. It didn't help when the camera crew started following us around. It was a whirlwind. Soph was oblivious to it all. After our day of filming, she slept through the night for the first time ever.

The official trade period only went for a few days, but it felt like much longer. It was intense. There was a lot of back and forth between the Giants and Port. Jeremy wasn't being poached; he was *asking* to be poached. It's hard to be traded on your own terms. Port wasn't looking for a tall forward, but we were offering one up. In the end, Jeremy was traded for a Round 3 pick. Port signed Jezz for the remaining two years he had on his Giants contract, plus a third year. And all they traded in return was a Round 3 pick. The Giants did the right thing by us, having realised how much we needed to be on home soil.

Some people—especially those on Facebook—couldn't believe the Giants had let Jezz go, and for such a small trade, too. The thing was, Jeremy hadn't played the last four games of that year's season. The reason he hadn't played was because he was having a baby and didn't want to be stranded on the other side of the country, but that didn't matter on the spreadsheet. The stats showed Jeremy had been absent for four rounds and, as such, he was dispensable. The Giants' loss was Port's gain.

Jeremy's new team rented us a townhouse near the club to settle into. I stayed in Port Lincoln while Jezz got things organised and waited for our furniture to arrive from the east coast. He was sleeping on a blow-up mattress from Bunnings, sitting on a plug-in cooler that doubled as his fridge, eating microwave meals and watching TV on my laptop. Oh, the glamour.

But it didn't matter to us. Jeremy was stoked to be training with his new club and getting stuck in. And I was glad to be home. I was going to be an Adelaide girl again. I was going to raise my daughter, and cheer on my partner, in my home state. I couldn't have been happier.

~

My first job, at sixteen, was working behind the counter at an Adelaide shopping-centre bakery. Two of my friends worked there as well. There was a cheesemonger across from us, so we'd swap them sourdough for brie and eat like kings every break. I lived off the olive sourdough and an assortment of cheeses during that time.

I had moved to Adelaide on my own to do Year 11 and 12 at Sacred Heart College. Well, that was the story, but let's be real: I did it for a boy. My high school boyfriend Jed (another J!) had gone away to boarding school in Adelaide and I planned to join him. But before I started at the boarding school, I was caught trying to get my phone charger from Jed's room—and, naturally, I was banned from the boarding house.

I was lucky, though. My mum's biological mother lived in Adelaide, so I stayed with her for the first three months. Eventually I moved into a little unit that was similar to university accommodation. There was a bus stop right out the front, so I'd catch the bus to school every day. I was living on my own, going to school, playing sport and working part-time at the bakery to support myself. I ate frozen meals or avocado on toast for dinner every night, plus the aforementioned olive sourdough at the bakery. It's lucky I was sporty because I made friends quickly, and lucky I was studious because otherwise I could have run wild. I had my provisional licence, once I'd turned seventeen, and a little car, so I really could do whatever I wanted.

It was a big move—leaving the sticks for the big city at age sixteen—but it was the best thing I could've done for myself. I was already used to standing on my own two feet, but the move made me stand up taller. It really instilled my sense of independence.

When I finished high school, I stayed in Adelaide, moving into a share house with my boyfriend and his brother and his brother's girlfriend. I was studying teaching at university, with the aim of becoming a high school maths teacher. I knew teaching was something I could do anywhere, and maths was a universal language. I wanted to go places in life, and teaching would give me opportunities to do just that.

I was twenty when I went through the hardest thing I'd experienced in my life to that point. I got a call in the early hours of the morning. My uncle had had a heart attack in his sleep and died. I got the call because I was the oldest cousin (by one year), and was tasked with breaking the news to my cousin that her dad had died. It was 2 a.m. when I drove the 30 minutes to my cousin's place. When I rocked up on her doorstep, I was a mess.

'What did he do?' my cousin asked, thinking I'd had a fight with my boyfriend.

I broke down. I couldn't form words, let alone sentences.

'No, it's Paul,' I managed to get out.

'Who the fuck is Paul?' my cousin asked, not used to using her dad's first name.

'He's dead. Your dad's gone,' I said. I didn't know what else to say. There were no words. I held my cousin as the news sunk in. It was devastating. My uncle was only 55 years old. He was too young. It wasn't right.

Little did I know, it wouldn't be the last hard thing I'd go through.

~

One week Jeremy was making a joke about me needing a portaloo. The next, I was told I had bowel cancer. After Jeremy called her on the way home from the hospital to tell her the news, my mum booked the next flight from Port Lincoln to Adelaide. She told me that the night before her morning flight was the longest she'd ever experienced. *We're meant to keep our children safe and healthy,* my mum kept thinking. *My daughter has cancer. I want to fix it for her, but I don't know how.*

The day after my diagnosis, I walked into my surgeon's office. His name was Dr G and he was a fabulous man in his forties.

'We're going to cure you,' Dr G said after he introduced himself. 'Obviously we don't know the extent of the disease yet, but you're young, fit and healthy, and you have a purpose.' He pointed to Sophia. 'We're going to fight this,' Dr G continued. I liked him right away.

The surgeon and his assistant, Emily, explained what was going to happen. Or at least they tried to. When Dr G realised his words were going in one of my ears and out the other, he started drawing diagrams for me. It helped me wrap my head around the surgery I was staring down. The operation was called a colostomy. Essentially, it would divert my bowels to my stomach to eliminate the risk of a bowel obstruction, since the tumour was going to continue growing before it shrank with the chemo and radiotherapy.

When the time came for questions, I only had one: 'What happens with my fertility?'

I knew if the treatment was going to involve chemotherapy, I would lose my fertility. I'd just had a baby and I knew I wanted more. I was desperate to keep my fertility at all costs.

'You've got a daughter,' Dr G said.

'Yes, but what about the future? I want to give her siblings,' I pressed.

The look on his face told me more than his words. The surgeon asked me if I'd had my period since giving birth, and I told him I wasn't really sure. I didn't think so.

'Normally, to do an egg retrieval for future IVF, you need to have had your period,' he explained.

'Well, can you try to get some eggs anyway?' I pushed.

'You have a surgery in five days,' he said.

He was trying to tell me I didn't have time to go through the process of an egg retrieval, without telling me that I was out of time.

I kept pushing the issue, and Dr G gave me the number for a fertility specialist, but he made it clear that egg retrieval wasn't going to be likely in my case. Oh, and he also told me

I had to wean my three-month-old daughter off breastmilk in the next three days.

That was a brutal truth to process. *How will I feed my daughter? She doesn't go to sleep with a bottle. How will she survive? I'll never be able to breastfeed again. How will I survive?*

I spiralled. Mum tried to talk me off the ledge. 'It's okay. Sophia takes a bottle. She'll be fine on formula,' she reasoned.

'I suggest you go cold turkey, because otherwise you're going to be in hospital and you'll still be producing milk and unable to get rid of it,' Dr G advised. 'I suggest you go home tonight and do what you need to do, then switch to bottles tomorrow.'

He made it sound simpler than it was.

I nursed Sophia to sleep that night, and in the morning I expressed my milk in the shower. That was it. We started alternating between the breastmilk I had stored and formula. Naturally, Sophia only liked the most expensive formula, even though we tried many different types.

In truth it was harder for me than her, which gave me some comfort. So too did this: as much as I lost, Jeremy gained. Being able to feed our baby gave him a whole new purpose. He was able to bond with Sophia in an entirely new way. They developed a special connection.

Everything I knew to be motherhood was put on pause, I was weaning my daughter and myself off breastfeeding, while processing the news that I'd have no time to harvest my eggs in hopes of extending our family with my own biology, and to top off the list of things I'd rather not have to do, I also had the task of telling my loved ones about my diagnosis. My close friends were absolutely shattered. Kobi was physically sick when I called her and broke the news. She sounded as confused as I felt, and asked a million questions. 'How? Why? What does that mean? What's next?' she asked. 'What about Soph?'

It was a common reaction. Jeremy's sister-in-law, Jess, couldn't believe it. 'My heart sank,' she told me later. 'When you hear "cancer", you naturally think "death". I was also angry. How could this beautiful time of being new parents be ripped from you and Jeremy? And Sophia? You didn't deserve it.'

No one knew what to say or do. Seeing my friends' reactions made it all the more real, and really fucking scary. There was less shock and more sadness. I could see the immense fear on their faces, and I found myself constantly assuring them that I would be okay. As soon as I said that, they'd agree wholeheartedly. 'If anyone is going to get through, it's you, Kell,' they said. I hoped they were right.

There are so many things I can look back on as silver linings. But hindsight can still be a bitch. I have thought about what would have happened if I'd had the colonoscopy that was cancelled in 2020. Yes, they would have found the tumour sooner, but I wouldn't have had Sophia. Without Sophia, I wouldn't have had the same purpose: to live. To raise my baby. To do whatever it takes. My daughter gave me the strength to survive. If it wasn't for her, I wouldn't be writing this book right now.

4

Dot, dot, dot

I know you're not supposed to google medical things, but I couldn't help myself. I was sitting in my surgeon's rooms waiting to have a colostomy operation when I googled 'what do stomas look like?' The images that popped up were confronting and a bit frightening: red, puckered and angry.

Scrolling through the images, it was hard to imagine having one on my body, but that's what I was there to get. A stoma is a surgically created opening on the abdomen that allows bowel movements to leave the body into a bag. I needed one because the obstruction in my bowel was so large, I couldn't pass anything through it. The threat of sepsis was real, so a colostomy was needed. To create a stoma, the end of the bowel is brought out through the opening and stitched onto the skin. In simple terms, it's a makeshift bumhole on your tummy.

To prepare me for the surgery, my stoma nurse, Paula, showed me a little rubber model of what my stoma would look like. Even with the model stuck to my side, I couldn't imagine having one. But I didn't have time to get my head around it; things were happening quicker than I could process them. From the moment the gastroenterologist showed me a photo of my bowel and said, 'This is what bowel cancer looks like,' there was a never-ending whirlwind of appointments, tests and scans. And then, on 25 November, my first surgery: a colostomy.

I have friends who live with Crohn's disease. Recently they told me about their fear of being fitted with a colostomy bag. Before every surgery, they say the same thing to their doctors: 'If you have to put a bag on, don't wake me up.'

I'm glad I didn't know that before my colostomy surgery.

Other than the grommets surgery I had when I was a few weeks old, the colostomy was the first surgery I'd had—unless extraction of my wisdom teeth counted. For some reason I wasn't scared of the procedure, just the outcome. I'd been sedated before—I knew how good it felt to wake up from an anaesthetic, and I was almost looking forward to that part. Just as I was about to go under, my surgeon called out to my anaesthetist to 'push the Michael Jackson juice'. I felt comfort in knowing Dr G would be the one operating on me. I'd grown to love him—the man who literally had my life in his hands—faster than you'd probably expect. His bedside manner was impeccable. So too was his ability to relate to me as his patient, regardless of the fact that I was 50-plus years younger than the patients he was used to.

The surgery itself only took an hour, but the preparation beforehand took 24 hours, and it didn't fully work: when I arrived, we discovered that there was a bowel obstruction and my bowels weren't as empty as the prep should have made them. Dr G was probably stressed, but he didn't show it.

When I woke up, I was already in the ward. I must have slept through my time in the recovery room. I was in pain. I had four incisions, including the hole the size of a 5-cent piece where my stoma had been created. The other three were tiny little 2–5 millimetre incisions—all that had been needed for the keyhole procedure. It seemed crazy to me: this man had performed major surgery with only the tiniest of entry points.

I managed the pain with my good friend fentanyl, which I became well acquainted with over the next few months. The worst aspect of the pain was the gas trapped in my chest. For the surgeons to see clearly, they need to expand your abdominal area with gas—which doesn't always escape before you're stitched up, and it takes a few days for your body to get rid of it. I couldn't even sit up without being in excruciating pain, not from anything other than this trapped gas. I figured if that was the worst of my problems, I'd done well. Paula checked on me every hour or so, making sure I was okay. They had a clear bag on the stoma so the nurses could easily see if there was any activity, which meant I could also see the stoma any time I moved my blanket. This took *a lot* to get used to. It was foreign, it was a bumhole on my stomach, it was not something any 25-year-old would want.

At the time, I felt like my life was falling apart, but now I can see how lucky I was. I wasn't alone in being a young person with a stoma. I've since met several people with them and you'd never know they had one. The reality is, a colostomy bag is a necessary and helpful medical device. It's not the gross little poo bag you might manifest in your mind.

My stoma was smaller than I imagined, but it still freaked me out. Some people name their stoma to form some connection with it, but I didn't want to get attached. I hoped it was only going to be temporary. There would be no name for my stoma.

There would be rules, though. I was warned not to eat corn because the kernels would come out whole in my bag. I couldn't run or play rough sports. I had to learn how to clean my stoma and change my colostomy bag—Paula showed me some tips and tricks to make it easier. She also reminded me that stomas are for output only, they are not a new hole to experiment with—which provided a much-needed laugh in such an overwhelming environment. I learned really quickly that laughing does in fact limit the crying. The hardest thing was not being allowed to lift Sophia up because I would get a hernia.

I knew it was for the greater good. Having a colostomy bag would make things much easier for me when I started treatment, and it would also give me the ability to have bowel movements again. What a treat. I tried to look on the bright side. I played a fun game where I timed how long it would take a cup of coffee to go through me. (It was twenty minutes FYI.)

I cracked jokes, but I was still self-conscious. A lot of people shower without their bag—so their stoma is showing—but I was quite protective of mine. I've never let Jeremy see it, or my parents or Sophia. My dad didn't even know that it was a piece of my bowel until months after I'd had it reversed. He thought there was a medical tube sticking out of me, not my literal bowels stitched to my abdomen.

I didn't want anyone to see it if they didn't have to. It's something you can't unsee. This might sound vain, but I didn't want Jeremy picturing my stoma when he closed his eyes to kiss me. Because of that, I changed my bag and cleaned my stoma on my own. I turned my home office into my stoma room, and I kept all my cleaning supplies and refills in Sophia's old changing table. I had a mirror and bin in there so I could do everything by myself. It was my way of trying to protect my loved ones from the gruesomeness of what I was going through.

My mum immediately came to live with us in Adelaide after I was diagnosed. She's always been the person I could turn to when I needed something—in high school she was that person for all my mates, too—and this was no exception. I needed my mum. My daughter needed my mum. Jeremy *really* needed my mum. We would've been utterly lost without her.

I was told I had to stay in hospital for a week after my surgery. Sophia couldn't enter the hospital because, at three months old, she couldn't be vaccinated for Covid-19. We applied for an exemption given Sophia's age prevented her from being able to comply with the regulations, but that was going to take time. I could appreciate that these regulations were in place for a good reason—if Sophia was exposed to Covid she could be at a heightened risk—but the risks were far outweighed by the intense need to be with my baby and strong feeling that she needed to be with me, too. One of the managers at the hospital understood what I was going through and was good about Sophia visiting, but when she wasn't working we didn't know if we were going to get into trouble having her there. One time, I told a nurse I was going downstairs to get a coffee from the cafe, and I actually snuck out into the hospital carpark to see Soph. Another time, Mum literally put Sophia in her jacket and smuggled her into my recovery room. I don't know how we thought we'd pulled that one off, the nurses definitely chose not to say anything when they saw exactly what was going on, but it was the greatest gift Mum had ever given me. I couldn't pick Sophia up or hold her normally because I was in pain and couldn't move properly, but just seeing her was special. Mum laid her down in between my legs on the hospital bed, and then propped her up on a pillow so I could feed her with a bottle. Being able to feed my baby felt like a triumph.

It was a Saturday when I was allowed to go home—only three days after my surgery rather than the week they had initially said. I had a week to recover in my own space and get ready for the next phase of treatment. I needed to wake my bowels up and make sure everything with my stoma was working. My bowels saw the surgery as an attack, so paralysed themselves and went to sleep. I started forcing water and food down, trying to get some movement happening.

I was staring down a gruelling few months. First up, I'd do five weeks of radiotherapy and oral chemotherapy, then I'd get a break. Then six rounds of intravenous chemo. The idea was to shrink the cancer as much as possible before undergoing surgery to remove it.

While I was having my colostomy operation, Dr G took a biopsy of the tumour. I met with him on a Monday morning to get the lay of the land. His tone had changed. When I first met him, he said, 'We're going to cure you. We're going to fight this.' On that Monday, he said, 'We're going to try to prolong your life.'

There Must Be More

It wasn't the words that knocked me, it was the shift in energy. The other people in the room—Emily, Jeremy, Mum and Jess—were quiet. Dr G had been so confident in the beginning, and he'd lost some of that assurance. Naturally, my outlook took a hit because of that.

I was glad I had already wrapped my head around what was to come. All I had to do was get through the next six weeks of treatment, and then the six weeks after that. There was a plan and I held onto it like a life raft. So many things were out of my control, but I could control what was immediately in front of me.

First thing, I needed to get tatted up. I had to have three tiny dots tattooed on my lower abdomen as a part of the radiotherapy planning. A nurse used a scalpel to make two marks on each of my hips and one right in the middle, then she painted the indents with ink. The dots would help line the radiation machine up to make sure the treatment was accurate. They were going to send radiation beams into my body to destroy the cancer cells, so naturally they wanted to fry the right spot.

The tiny tattoos were a sign of the uncertainty I was facing. What was to come? Who knew. Dot, dot, dot.

~

'Mum! I got a tattoo!' I was calling home from a holiday in Europe. 'It's a J, in my own handwriting. I got it for Jed.'

Jed, my high school sweetheart, and I had very recently broken up.

'You what!?' Mum lost it.

I let her panic for a moment before telling her the truth. 'I'm only joking, Mum. It's for you, Dad and Jake,' I explained, admiring the new ink on my tiny bicep. I thought my joke was hilarious. Mum? Not so much.

I met Jed at an athletics carnival when I was thirteen. He was a year older than me and lived an hour and a half from Port Lincoln, in a town called Cleve. He was an attractive young lad, and there weren't many of those in our neck of the woods. All the girls used to swoon over him at the sports carnivals. Somehow, I managed to get his Snapchat—as you did in those days—and we started messaging. Jed was a total boy's boy, but I found out he was also a big softie.

One weekend, a year or so later, Jed came to Port Lincoln for a local footy carnival, and we went to the movies to see *Kung Fu Panda* with a few friends. Somehow Jed and I ended up sitting next to each other. And *somehow* his hand ended up on top of mine. We had a hug at the end of the movie, and it was a massive deal. We were on.

From that day on, Jed and I were besotted. Every second weekend I'd make Mum drive me to Cleve after my A-grade netball game so I could see him. Poor Mum would have to drive all the way back the next day to pick me up. Most of the time, there'd be three of my friends in the car with Mum when she came to get me. 'Oh, we were just walking past your house when your mum was getting in the car, so we thought we'd come for a drive,' they would explain. Everyone loved my mum.

I did, too, and I also fell in love with Jed's family. They were all beautiful, and I became very close with his mum, Kylie.

At school in Adelaide, Jed and I were almost like a golden couple. Because we were both from the Eyre Peninsula and both into sports, our friendship groups were intertwined. We did everything together. Even when we were hanging out with our friends, we'd be doing it together. Our mates would call us 'Mum and Dad' because we were in a solid relationship, not the usual three-month fling common in high school.

After school, we moved into our share house, and Jed became a builder and was working on construction sites while I went to uni to study teaching.

As a kid I thought I'd be a nurse or a midwife, but my fear of needles and inability to look at blood put an end to that. Still, I had a desire to help, and that's what led me to teaching. I knew being a teacher would allow me to care for others, to protect them and to help them become better. I also knew that teaching was a degree that could take me anywhere.

I majored in sport and maths at university. With Mum being an accountant, numbers were in my DNA. I studied a year ahead in maths for all of high school, so I finished Year 12 maths when I was in Year 11. It was my strong suit—I was shit at English, couldn't write an essay to save myself and had a very limited vocabulary—so maths it was.

The first time I left Australia was on a family holiday to Bali as a kid. Such a cliché, I know, but it was a life-changing trip for me. It stirred something inside me. I felt a pull to travel.

Jed, on the other hand, wanted to put down roots. He had plans to build a house of his own and stay in South Australia. I wanted to get out of South Australia and travel the world. Our horizons looked very different.

We started bickering. It was clear we were moving in different directions, but neither of us wanted to say that out loud. After three or four months of uneasiness, it all came to a head in a disagreement over something trivial. Something had to give, and in the end, it was me. I packed my bags and left.

We were together for six years, and then we weren't. I was only just 21. We blocked and deleted each other, and I haven't spoken to Jed since then. I've bumped into his parents and brothers out and about in Adelaide, but I've never run into him. It's like we move in entirely different circles these days. Which is so strange for little old Adelaide.

Jed was a big part of my life. If it weren't for him, I wouldn't have moved to Adelaide on my own at sixteen, and

I wouldn't have become the person I am today. That move was essentially the start of my life.

~

I started chemo and radiotherapy on my 26th birthday, 6 December 2021. It sounds like a shitty way to spend your birthday, but it was actually okay. Because I hadn't started taking the treatment yet, I was fine the morning of my birthday and I got to spend it with Jeremy, Sophia and my mum. My dad and brother came to Adelaide, too; it was the first time they'd seen me since my diagnosis.

It was a weird feeling. No one knew how to act around me. *I* didn't even know how to act around me. Everything was unknown, and the only thing we thought we knew was that a cancer diagnosis was a death sentence. I can only imagine the thoughts my family were all having but not expressing. I wanted normality and everyone around me wanted that, too, so we went on as if it were nothing. But it wasn't nothing.

At the hospital, the nurses gave me the side effects run-down—and a box of chocolates for my birthday. It was so sweet. What came next wasn't, though.

I was warned I could get burn marks on my skin from where the radiation hit. The radiation would also make me extremely sensitive to the sun. And the chemo could make me nauseous, fatigued and sore, and give me thrush.

I'd never seen a radiation machine before, then suddenly I was lying in a hospital bed underneath one. The nurse lined the machine up with my tattooed dots and the process began. It took less than five minutes. The machine spun one way for a minute and then the other for another. It rotated around me twice, and then it was done.

'Is that it?' I asked.

'That's it,' the nurse replied.

That was easy, I thought to myself. *I just lay there! I can do that for six weeks, no trouble.*

Oh, how naive I was.

The oral chemo was a lower dose than the intravenous chemo, but the consistency was aggressive because of the nature of my cancer. The pills were tiny, but they were toxic. Anyone touching them had to wear gloves. As soon as I started taking them, *I* became toxic. I had to be careful about everything I touched. I couldn't hug Jeremy or cuddle Sophia because it would have made them sick. I had a packet of Dettol wipes in the bathroom to wipe down any surfaces that I touched. I washed the shower after I used it, and flushed the toilet twice.

I had to be careful of what I came into contact with, and what came into contact with me. It was December 2021 and Covid was still spreading. Because of the chemo and radiotherapy, my immune system was dangerously vulnerable. I knew I couldn't get sick—not just because my body couldn't handle it, but also because I wouldn't be allowed to continue the treatment if I had Covid. The treatment was the only thing killing the cancer. I needed it.

Initially, at the time of my first colonoscopy, my cancer was graded as Stage 3, but after a PET scan in the week leading up to my colostomy surgery, the diagnosis was changed. The cancer had spread from my bowel, up my spine and throughout my abdomen. There were also spots on my lung. I was Stage 4. There's no Stage 5. My cancer was terminal.

This time, I didn't google what Stage 4 meant. I could handle seeing photos of stomas, but I couldn't handle being told I was going to die. I didn't want to know the statistics. I didn't want to count my days. I didn't want to face reality.

I blindsided myself.

5

Baby's first Christmas

Jeremy and I had never had a serious fight. Sure, we'd had disagreements and tiffs, but we never fought. My cancer changed that.

A few weeks into my treatment—two days before Christmas, 2021—we got into the biggest fight of our relationship.

I'd been putting on a brave face as much as I could. I knew Jezz and my family were going through so much already. They cried every day. I would come downstairs to find Jeremy and Mum in tears, and then I'd walk straight back upstairs. I couldn't bear to see them crying, and there was no way I was going to let them see *me* cry. Some days I'd be sobbing in bed, but as soon as someone else walked in the room, I'd wipe my eyes, roll over and act fine. It was like I was a character in a movie. In the movie, my character was fine: she was strong; she was going to be okay. I learned how to switch my character on and off in an instant. I committed to the role. I swear I could've snagged a part on *Home and Away*.

The truth was, I was scared.

Just like with my stoma, I hid the reality from everyone. Because of the nature of the pandemic, no one was allowed to come with me for my treatment at the hospital—I was there on my own—so no one heard the urgency in the nurses' voices as they read me the riot act. 'You cannot get Covid. You have to be so careful,' they drilled into me.

I tried to relay the message to everyone at home, but my voice mustn't have had as much authority as the nurses'.

On the outside, I didn't look sick. I still had my hair and I looked like myself. On the inside, though, my body was in fight mode. I was severely immunocompromised and the threat of Covid loomed heavily over me. Being exposed to Covid would literally be a life-or-death situation for me. And yet, I couldn't get that through to Jeremy.

It was summer and the Christmas holidays, so I understood everyone wanted to be out and about socialising. I would never have stopped Jeremy from doing that, but I did ask him—and everyone who was going to be in contact with me—to stick to outside venues. That was the advice at the time to avoid spreading the disease. It was a simple rule and I didn't think it was too much to ask for.

Our good friends Zac (yes, the bloke who was the first to know about baby Sophia) and Rachel were visiting us in

Adelaide over the holidays. It was 23 December, and Jezz and Zac decided to go to the pub. They picked one with an outside beer garden, so it was fine by me. I was at home with Rachel, Mum and Sophia. When we called the boys to check in, they didn't answer. I opened the Find My Friends app, and it looked like they were inside the pub. Not outside, as per our agreement.

I lost my shit. I had never felt so upset with Jeremy. I was furious at him for putting my health at risk by being inside a busy pub, but Jeremy thought I was angry because he'd been in the pokies room. He got defensive and tried to minimise the situation. 'I never play the pokies. It was just a little slap, not a big deal.'

I blew up.

'You don't understand,' I said. 'If you pick up Covid from inside the pub and give it to me, I can't continue my cancer treatment. This treatment is the only thing keeping me here.'

I was inconsolable. Mum said she'd never seen me like that before. She understood why I was fuming, but she was still taken aback at the steam coming out of my ears.

The tension was heavy. And my reaction was a reality check. Obviously, Jeremy wasn't thinking when he went inside the pub. He didn't realise the severity of the situation because he hadn't had to face it yet. Maybe he didn't fully comprehend it because I had shielded him from so much. It took my wrath to make him realise just how serious it was. It was an eye-opening experience for everyone.

The next day I was still mad, so I made Zac drive me to the hospital for treatment instead of Jeremy. Zac's sister also had cancer, so he understood more than most.

My blow-up made everything feel more real to me. Up until then, I don't think it had properly hit home yet. I mean, I understood I had cancer, but I hadn't yet fully grasped the gravity of the situation. It took an almighty argument to put things in focus. For me, and everyone around me.

After our first official row, Jeremy and I celebrated our baby's first-ever Christmas. For obvious reasons, it wasn't the day I had dreamed it would be.

In some ways, though, it was even better.

Our friends Sam and Izzy Jacobs, whom we got to know really well when Jeremy was playing with Sam at the Giants, were going away for Christmas. They offered us their home in Adelaide to stay in, to give us a bit more space. They had a five-bedroom, three-bathroom house with a big backyard and a pool. My parents and brother came to stay with us in the house, and Zac and Rachel stayed in our townhouse. It meant a lot to me to have my people around me.

After nearly three weeks of treatment, the fatigue had hit. I worked out I needed to have treatment in the morning, not the afternoon, because otherwise I'd spend all day feeling anxious about the appointment. I needed to rip the bandaid off. I would have radiotherapy at 9 a.m. and go home for a nap, and then I'd be able to function that afternoon.

I was warding off the nausea with anti-nausea tablets, but I still had to force myself to take my chemo medication every day. When you feel like shit, the last thing you want to do is swallow something that's going to make you feel more shit. Regardless, I was diligent about taking my tablets. And so was Mum.

Even when I was a kid, Mum didn't often tell me what to do. She didn't need to; I was pretty self-sufficient. So, it was a hard pill to swallow—figuratively and literally—when she had to parent me when I was an adult. I'd always prided myself on my independence, so losing that was tough. Mum hated it as much as I did. She didn't want to baby me, but she had to. Each morning Mum would bring me my chemo pill on a tray, like she was delivering me breakfast in bed. 'Room service,' she'd joke. It wasn't funny, but we had to laugh—it was the only way we could get through it.

~

'Mum, you've got to take me to the hospital!' I insisted. I was eleven and I was sure I was dying. I was bleeding, and it wasn't the first time. Fun fact: when I was younger, my mum had explained to me that I had been born with an irregular-sized kidney that didn't function. So, when I started bleeding, my first thought was, 'It's my kidney! I'm going to die!'

The first two times it happened, I kept the bleeding a secret from my mum—which was weird, because I never hid anything from her. She was the kind of mum you'd confide in. All my mates loved my mum. She would drive us to our netball training sessions and games and put up with six girls screaming and singing the whole way. She blames us for her deafness now. As we got older, Mum was the person we'd call to pick us up from parties. I knew I could talk to her about anything, even awkward things, but I chose not to talk to her about this.

It wasn't until the bleeding happened a third time that I knew there was something seriously, terribly wrong with me. I made Mum take me to the hospital because I was sure I was sick.

I told the nurse my symptoms. I was bleeding 'down there' and had an ache in my tummy. For the third time in three months!

'Um, she's got her period,' the nurse explained.

'I know,' Mum replied. 'Can you tell her that? She's not listening to me.'

Once I wrapped my head around the concept of menstruation, I grabbed a tampon and got on with things. Crisis averted. Phew. I was still in primary school and the first of my friends to get their period, so I made sure to tell all my mates not to worry if they started bleeding. I'd tell them what to do.

I wasn't dying, but I could have died from embarrassment. Who goes to the hospital for their period? I realised I'd completely overreacted and felt silly. It was a teachable moment. I learned you only go to the hospital for emergencies. I learned if something didn't feel right, I was probably overreacting. I learned I should just suck it up and get on with things.

I learned the wrong lesson.

~

On Christmas Day I plastered a smile on my face, but under my mask, I was wrecked. Because it was a holiday, I had the day off from treatment. I was relieved not to have to do radiation, but then I felt anxious because I wasn't doing radiation. Boxing Day was a public holiday, too, so I wasn't being treated for two days. I was worried what that might mean for the cancer. As much as I was grateful for the little break from the radiation beams, it was almost harder for me without them. I knew I could physically cope with the treatment, but without it, I felt unsure.

We woke up on Christmas Day to open presents with Sophia. She was mesmerised by the wrapping paper, as four-month-olds are, and didn't pay too much attention to the actual gifts. Her presents were mostly practical things, such as a pool floaty, fruit teethers, clothes and the odd noisy toy.

Zac and Rachel came over and we all wore matching festive pyjamas. It was really sweet. Even more so when Zac surprised me with my first Louis Vuitton. What!? He assured me I deserved it. I was over the goddamn moon.

After unwrapping the presents under the tree, I was exhausted. 'Go have a nap,' Jeremy suggested.

'I don't want to miss out!' I told him. I wanted to push through. It was my daughter's first Christmas; I didn't want to sleep the day away.

As the morning went on, everyone migrated outside to the pool, as you do on Christmas Day Down Under. But the sun was out, and that meant I couldn't be. As I mentioned, because of the radiotherapy, I was extremely sensitive to the sun, and I couldn't spend more than ten minutes out in it. The nurses had told me I needed to be really careful, and I did as I was told. Normally I'd be in a little bikini soaking up the vitamin D, but I was so scared of exposing my skin, I wore a full-piece swimsuit with bike shorts on top to give me an extra layer of material over the area the radiation was targeting. In my get-up, I quickly jumped in and out of the water and returned to the shade. I was conscious of the sun, and also my stoma, which I was still pedantic about keeping clean and self-conscious of showing.

Sophia had her first swim on her first Christmas Day. It wasn't with me. I watched from afar as Rachel took her into the pool and played with her, jumping around, dunking her under the water and holding her up in the air. Soph had a ball and was an instant water baby. It was a beautiful moment, and I was so happy for Rach and Soph to share that special memory together, but I couldn't help feeling like I'd missed out on a milestone.

Fuck, I wish I could be in there, I thought to myself, watching my daughter splash happily in the pool. I was determined not to miss out on precious moments if I could help it, but there were some things I just couldn't risk.

After Christmas I had another two days off treatment for New Year's Day. Jeremy's brother, Nick, and Nick's wife, Jess, were in Adelaide visiting her family. They stayed an extra week so we could do something together to ring in the new year—although they knew we obviously couldn't have a rager.

We decided to go to Murray Bridge, an hour east of Adelaide. Naturally, everything was booked out, so we booked a one-bedroom cabin—the only accommodation that was available—and Nick and Jess stayed in their campervan. I had treatment on 30 December, and we left straight from the hospital. Mum came with us—and slept on the pull-out couch, bless her—to help with Sophia. There were four of us in the tiniest studio I've ever seen. It was nice and cosy. Any wonder Jezz wanted to get out and about.

On our first night at the river, Jeremy decided he wanted to go bowling. For the same reason I didn't want to sit inside at a cafe or pub, I didn't want to go to a bowling alley and run the risk of catching something. It had been a week since I'd blown up at Jezz for going into the pokies room at the pub, and it felt like deja vu.

'Just come. It's a small town, you'll be fine,' everyone was saying as they were getting ready to leave.

'No, it's fine. I'll stay here with Sophia,' I insisted. (It wasn't fine.)

I was exhausted after treatment, and had missed my nap because of the drive to Murray Bridge. There was no way I was going bowling. But I also didn't want to sit at home by myself, either. I felt alone. I didn't tell anyone that, though. The last thing I wanted was to be a burden. I'd rather feel like shit on my own than put any pressure on the people around me. I would never have told Jezz directly that I didn't want him to go bowling, or ask him to stay home with me. But I found myself wishing I didn't *need* to say anything, that he would just *know* how much I needed him. The resentment grew within me. There was an edge of snarkiness to my voice. I could hear it, but Jeremy was oblivious. He's a man.

It wasn't just the bowling, obviously. So many things had been adding up and wearing me down. Every coffee I couldn't go for, every swim I couldn't enjoy, every activity I wasn't up for. Those things were constant reminders that I wasn't 'normal' anymore. I was sick.

I felt like I was constantly being reminded of what had been taken from me and what I was missing out on. Don't get me wrong, I knew I still had so much—I was lucky to be spending New Year's with my family and having a little break together—but it still sucked that I couldn't join in the festivities, or even have a glass of champagne to toast the new year.

'Can you at least stay up until midnight?' Jeremy asked me.

'Nope, it's nine p.m., I'm going to bed,' I said.

Still, I set an alarm for midnight and woke up to watch the fireworks. By 'watch the fireworks', I mean I stayed in bed and FaceTimed Jeremy so I could see the night sky through a screen. Then I went straight back to sleep. Happy New Year.

I woke up on the first day of 2022 feeling fantastic. Everyone else had a sore head. Not me. I felt quite smug about it, and suggested we go for a fish down at the river. We found a spot on the riverbank under some big shade trees. Because it was so shady, I felt comfortable going for a swim, so I got to take Sophia for her first swim in a river. I was stoked—and slightly terrified of swimming in the murky water. I was also conscious of keeping my stoma clean. It was a quick swim, but it was a milestone I could be part of. I clung on to it, the same way I clung on to Soph in the cloudy river water.

6

The long, dark night

The oncology ward at the private hospital was overflowing. There were so many patients needing chemotherapy they had to open up another room—a regular hospital room—and squeeze more chairs into it.

It was February 2022, and I'd arrived for my first day of intravenous chemo. When the nurse ushered me into the room I saw two older men and an older woman already hooked up to their machines having their treatment. I felt out of place.

'Take your pick,' the nurse said to me, waving at the remaining chairs.

'I cannot make any decisions today,' I told her. 'Please tell me where to sit.'

I settled into a chair at the front and braced myself for what was to come.

I'd finished my first six-week block of treatment—radiotherapy and oral chemo—on 8 January, after which I entered limbo land. The time between finishing treatment and being scanned to see the results was a blur of uncertainty.

As it happened, this time coincided with Jeremy's last free weekends before the AFL preseason officially kicked off. Mum offered to look after Sophia so we could spend a couple of nights in a hotel together and have some quality time. I don't know how 'quality' it was—I couldn't even kiss the bloke!—but we had a nice, relaxing few days.

I thought I would get to leave limbo land after my scan, but that wasn't the case. The tests showed there had been a reduction in the size of the tumour, but the doctor couldn't tell me much more than that. Because of the radiation, everything was still inflamed, so the results didn't accurately reflect what was going on inside me. The good news was that nothing internally had been extremely damaged, so I could continue having treatment.

My oncologist looked at my bloods and devised my next eighteen weeks of treatment. It would involve six rounds of intravenous chemotherapy, where the drugs would be given in liquid form through a drip inserted into one of my veins. This would be supplemented by more oral chemo.

I used to be deathly afraid of needles. It was a full-blown phobia. The first time I had to get a blood test, I was sweating and hyperventilating like wild. In reality, I know it's just a

The long, dark night

small prick—they usually don't even hurt!—but fear doesn't deal in reality. I thought all my exposure to needles during my treatment might have helped me to get over my phobia, but it only made it worse.

When the chemo nurse hooked me up to the machine, I had to look away from the needle as she inserted it into my arm. I was lucky they let me have Jeremy with me in the room because it was my first time and there was so much paperwork to fill out. The idea of having to go through the six-hour treatment on my own with no support felt brutal, but that was the reality for so many patients during that time. I wouldn't wish chemo on anyone, and I especially wouldn't wish it on anyone in the middle of an isolating pandemic.

Not having a hand to hold during chemo makes it all the more lonely.

After wincing my way through the needle, I was given a dose of steroids to help minimise the side effects. Next up was the anti-nausea medication and the antifungal drug for first timers on chemo. Then came the two-hour infusion. I felt okay during it all. It was honestly just like sitting in a chair giving blood. I lulled myself into a false sense of security. I thought because I hadn't had hideous side effects with the radiotherapy and oral chemo, maybe it would be the same with this treatment. In all the movies I'd seen with chemo machines, the patients always started vomiting as soon as they were hooked up. That didn't happen to me, so I hoped I was the exception to the rule.

I started chatting to the older woman next to me, who was in her sixties and wearing activewear. She explained this was her second type of treatment; the first one hadn't worked. Even so, she was upbeat, and she looked well. I know now looks can be deceiving.

'When I'm not here, I spend my days in the garden,' she said with a smile.

I was impressed with her attitude, and her hopefulness. The woman had been living with her diagnosis for a year and had high hopes because they'd caught the cancer early. It made me think: in a year's time I could be on the other side of this thing. At that point, I still hadn't looked into what Stage 4 meant. I was so naive.

I had never seen a chemo port before that first day in the oncology ward. I didn't even know what it was. So, I didn't know how to ask the woman next to me about the valve in her chest. While I had an IV inserted in my arm, she had a cord going into her chest. It looked like a charger plugged into a power point. When we got chatting, the woman explained she was going through immunotherapy, so I figured that's why our plug-ins were different. It wasn't until another session down the track that I learned what a port was and how it worked. Essentially, it's a small device that's attached to a vein (usually in the upper chest area) that allows blood to be drawn and drugs to be given without accessing your veins, which I came to learn chemotherapy absolutely ruins.

After my first intravenous chemo session, I went home and had pasta for dinner. The nurse had told me carbs would help me absorb the drugs. I took an anti-nausea tablet before I ate, and finished my bowl.

It was the last full meal I would eat in a while. When I woke up the next morning, I couldn't even drink water. Everything tasted like poison. I tried cordial but couldn't keep it down. Mum called me to come downstairs to take my morning tablets, but I couldn't get out of bed.

Mum was staying in one spare room, and Jeremy moved into the other because of my toxicity.

My hands had seized up like claws. I couldn't hold a knife and fork. I was numb to heat, and cold felt like fire. I couldn't tell that the shower water was boiling hot. It was terrifying. I didn't know what was happening to me. I was warned to expect side effects, but I didn't expect anything like this.

I had been told about neuropathy—which can happen after the type of chemo I'd received—but I didn't realise that's what I was experiencing. Neuropathy is a nerve condition that can lead to pain, numbness, weakness or tingling. The way it was explained to me, I thought that neuropathy just meant I couldn't drink cold water or touch the freezer walls. The reality was far more extreme.

I spiralled. I became too scared to eat or drink anything because food and drink tasted so toxic. By 4 p.m. I'd decided to call my surgeon's assistant and nurse, Emily, who had given me her number in case I needed anything. 'If the side effects keep occurring, go to the ER,' she told me.

The ER was the last place I wanted to go. I knew it was overrun at the best of times, let alone during a pandemic. I'd heard horror stories of people being left in triage rooms on their own, stuck without any way to call for help. Nope. I wasn't going. I held off. I curled up. I tried to uncurl my fingers.

At 10 p.m. I called Emily again (the poor woman; she never should have given me her number). I was desperate. I needed her help.

'You need to go to the ER,' she said.

'I'm not going to a public hospital,' I said. 'It's too risky.' I was afraid.

'Okay, if you can hold off until the morning, we can get you a bed in the private hospital,' she offered.

I deteriorated rapidly overnight. My temperature spiked and I started seizing up. I longed to sleep, but I couldn't. Nothing helped. Everything hurt. In the darkness, I genuinely thought I was going to die. I didn't think I would make it through the night.

In my mind, I debated whether it was better for me to tell Jeremy I was going to die, or for him to find my body in the morning. *How on earth do I tell Jeremy I'm not going to make it?* I thought to myself. The words didn't come.

When the morning came, somehow I was still alive. I felt like death, though. I could barely speak. I couldn't even look at my daughter. All I could look at was the back of my eyelids. A single thought repeated in my mind: *I can't do five more rounds of this. I can't do five more rounds of this.*

When I got to the hospital, I was so dehydrated my veins had collapsed. I was on the brink of collapse myself. Jeremy was able to drop me off and come into the hospital with me, but as soon as the nurses came in and started working on me, he had to leave.

I was all on my own.

~

Alone time didn't exist in my childhood. There were seven kids in our generation of cousins, as well as all of the family-by-choice 'cousins' we inherited. We were all pretty close in age, and went to the same primary school so there was always someone to hang out with in the school yard. Our family had a holiday home at Coffin Bay, on the other side of the peninsula, and we spent all our Christmases and Easters there with our aunties, uncles and cousins, at the beach, in the sun, under the water.

It sounds idyllic, and it was. My childhood was easy, contented, simple. I didn't have any major issues or losses growing up; I'm privileged in that sense.

I was still young when my grandma was diagnosed with breast cancer. She went to Adelaide for treatment and came back a few months later. She was fine. I knew cancer was a thing, but to me, it felt like it existed on the peripheral. It was real, but it was far away. Cancer was something that happened to other people. It wasn't something that would happen to me, I thought.

My biggest injury as a kid was a hairline fracture in one of my vertebrae. I slipped over in the school gymnasium and ended up in a neck and back brace for a few weeks. It wasn't the fracture that hurt the most, it was the whiplash. I'll never forget that feeling. It obviously hurt at the time, but in the grand scheme of things it wasn't that bad. I was a healthy, active kid, and I came from a healthy, active family. My mum managed all my sports teams (which was a workout of its own), and Dad and Jake were right into motocross sports.

Our house was always bustling with people: cousins, neighbours, friends. And pets. We always had animals: a border collie named Dylan who walked with a limp after jumping out of the tray of a ute and breaking his leg; a Maltese shih tzu named Marley with a hectic underbite; and another border collie, Benji, who knocked up another dog and gave us Louis.

The long, dark night

For my birthday one year, my best friend's family gave me a ragdoll cat from their litter. I cherished that animal like it was my baby. I named him Laker (because I was obsessed with basketball), and forbade my brother from touching him.

My dad was a cat dad. I think he liked them because they were less work for him. Dad was always up to something; his shed was a hive of activity. The shed was bigger than the house and it was Dad's pride and joy. It's all he ever wanted in life. In his shed, he's content.

I don't think my parents will ever leave Port Lincoln. It's all they know. Life is easy.

I don't think I could ever live there again. I also don't know if my life will ever be easy again.

∼

We didn't know it then—during my first round of intravenous chemo—but I was allergic to the oxaliplatin in the regime, and that's what gave me the neuropathy. The side effects of chemo are notoriously brutal, but what I was experiencing was more than that: it was an allergic reaction. I was in anaphylactic shock. My body was shutting down. My claw hands were a sign that the oxaliplatin was toxic to me. But my oncologist didn't pick up on it.

At the hospital, the morning after the night in which I was sure I was going to die, I was pumped full of nutrients and liquids. I was force-fed food, which was better than the alternative of having a nasal tube fitted. The nurses literally revived me. Within hours, I started to feel better. My claw hands slowly unfurled. I was lucky that nurse Emily was working at the hospital that day; she came to check on me. Seeing a familiar friendly face made all the difference.

I stayed in the hospital for three nights. When Jeremy and Mum came to visit me, I couldn't adequately explain what I was going through. They knew I felt like shit, but they didn't understand how severe it was. I couldn't understand it myself, and I was experiencing it.

'Have a drink of water,' they encouraged.

'I can't,' I replied. 'I honestly can't.'

They didn't get it. If I relented and had a sip of water to appease them, I would spew it back up.

It was the first time I truly thought, *Why me?* I'd been focused on doing what I had to do, but in that moment I felt defeated. It wasn't fair.

And yet, the show had to go on. The next time I went in for chemo, they stretched the infusion over four hours instead of two, to give my body more time to adjust. Then, I ended up in hospital three days later, instead of two.

The third time, I was admitted to hospital from the get-go. I was given a bed, and they did the infusion there. Again, I stayed for a few days because I was so unwell.

I was struggling with my third infusion when the first round of the 2022 AFL season kicked off in mid-March.

Four-year-old me—I'm starting to see more and more similarities between my daughter Sophia and my younger self as Soph approaches the same age.

Sport was always a huge part of my life. I met Eyerus Curtis in kindy when we were four and we've been friends since. Five years later we were together at the U12s Country Championships Basketball Carnival in our Port Lincoln Sharks basketball kits.

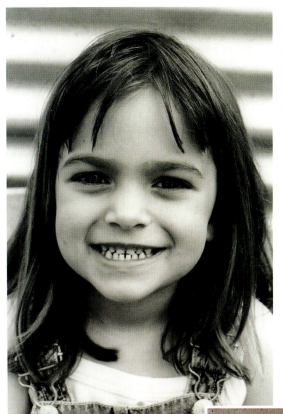

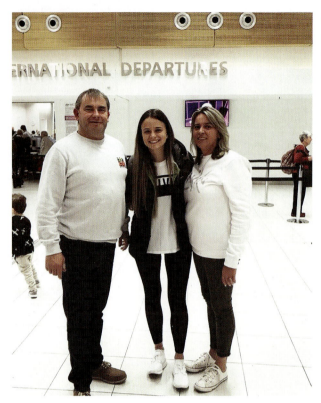

My parents saw me off to my teaching job in Norway at the departure gates in May 2018, and I was so excited for my new adventure.

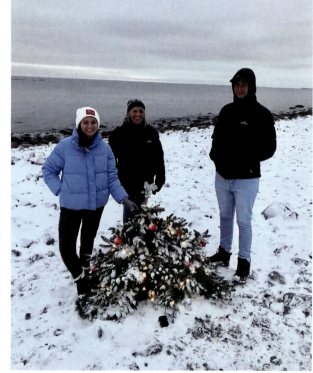

Mum and Jake met me in Norway for Christmas in 2018. For me and for Jake it was our first white Christmas; for Mum it was a chance to share a piece of herself with us as she had lived in Arendal as a teenager with her family.

Jake and I went to a church in Arendal on Christmas Eve, which is the day Scandinavians celebrate Christmas. The next day we were out on the slopes!

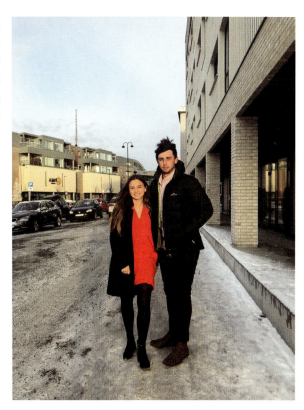

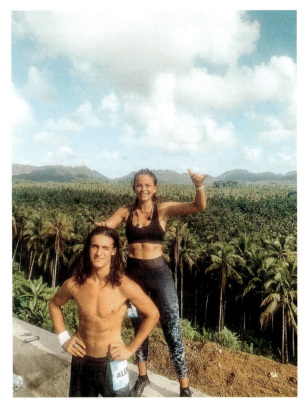

I ran my very first half marathon in Siargao in the Philippines with absolutely no training—the most I'd run before was 8 kilometres! I took this moment at the end for a victory shot with my friend Jack Allwood.

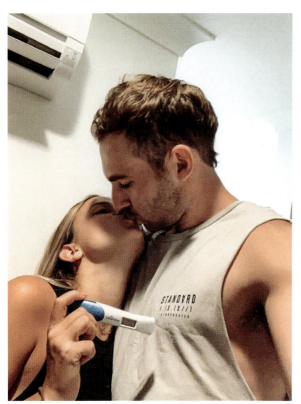

We were over the moon when we first discovered Sophia's existence, and she remains the highlight of our lives.

Sophia spent the first four days of her life in the NICU while the staff made sure she could regulate her temperature and blood sugars on her own and while we fell utterly and eternally in love with her.

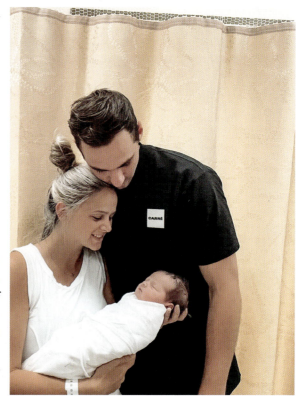

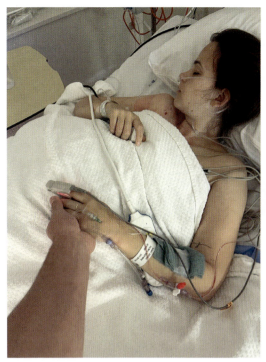
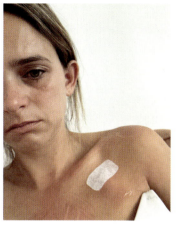

Left: After my ultra-low anterior resection, I was in the ICU. The only thing I remember is my neck hurting intensely.
Right: Ugly tears were necessary as I came to terms with my portacath completely ruining (in my opinion) my decolletage just weeks before getting married in a strapless dress. Sometimes it's unexpected small bumps that knock you down.

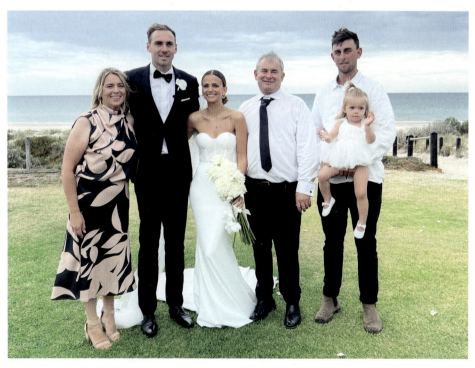

Mum, Dad, my brother Jake and Soph with Jezz and me on our wedding day in March 2023. A day I will never forget.

The game is on! Sophia and I joined Daddy in the Adelaide Oval rooms after a win in 2024. Our favourite part of the week is supporting Jezz at his games as much as we possibly can.

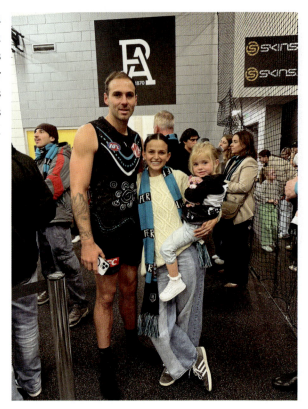

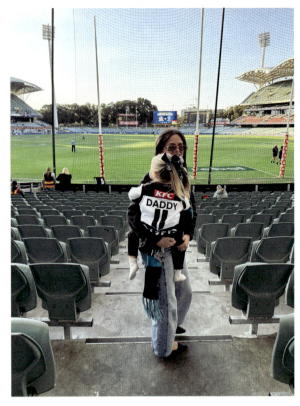

Me and Soph with her Daddy jumper on before a game. We go down behind the goals before every game and give Jezz a kiss, a cuddle and a high five for good luck while he warms up.

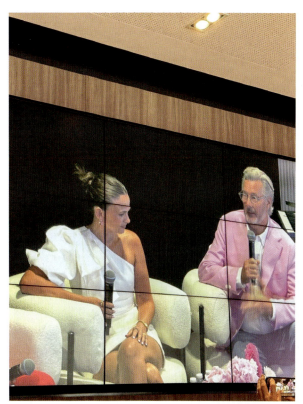

Barry Du Bois and I were a part of a panel for the 2024 McGrath Foundation High Tea in collaboration with Cricket Australia. They announced that their care was about to extend from breast cancer to all cancers.

In 2023 I became the face of the Jodi Lee Foundation 'Trust Your Gut' campaign. This campaign launched a fantastic online symptom checker to help people take first steps to care for their bodies.

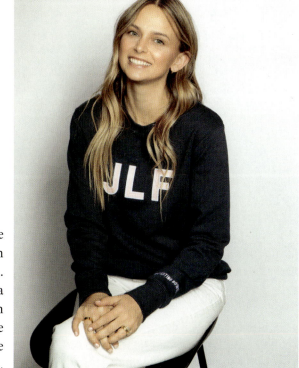

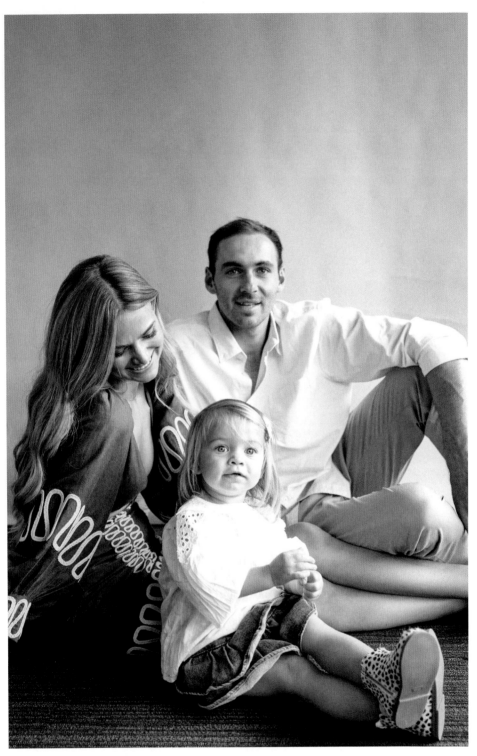

A family photo of Soph, Jezz and me—before I lost my hair. These two are the loves of my heart and the two strands of purpose anchoring me in my darkest hours.

The long, dark night

I watched the Carlton versus Richmond game on the couch. In the second quarter, Carlton player Sam 'Doc' Docherty kicked a goal from 30 metres out. It was a great kick, made even more extraordinary by the fact that Doc had undergone chemotherapy for testicular cancer in 2021. The goal brought down the house. The crowd roared from the stands and Doc's teammates mobbed him on the field.

I burst into tears. Of course I was happy for Doc, but the tears were also for myself. In a moment of self-pity, I thought, *If he could get through it, why can't I?*

After the third round, I had a PET scan to see how the treatment was working. I wasn't feeling hopeful.

'Do you want the good news or the bad news?' Dr G asked me.

'The bad news.' I wanted to rip off the bandaid.

'The bad news is, you're going to have to keep doing the chemo,' he said. 'The good news is, it's gone.'

'What's gone?' I asked.

'Nothing has shown up as active on the scan. It's gone,' he repeated.

It was some kind of miracle. Dr G explained he had another patient—a young bloke—on the exact same treatment plan as me. At his scan, the results showed his cancer had doubled in size. Whereas mine had responded so well to the treatment that there was no activity showing up. Sure, there was still a mass in my rectum that needed to be removed, but the metastasis that they were concerned about was gone.

Jeremy was at training when I messaged him the news. 'It's gone,' I wrote.

'What?' His reaction was the same as mine. Utter disbelief.

I should've been jumping for joy, but I was just too damn sick to move. There would be no jumping for me. The news should've made things easier; we knew the chemo was working. But it actually made it harder for me because I felt like I didn't have a reason to be doing it anymore. According to the scan, my cancer was gone, and I knew whatever was left of the tumour was going to be removed in a surgery. It felt like the chemo was killing me more than the cancer.

By my fifth chemo infusion, I was spent. I only managed to get halfway through the four-hour infusion before I started violently projectile vomiting all over the oncology ward. It went everywhere. I felt so terrible for the other patients in the room. Chemo makes you queasy enough, without having to see someone else be sick. I was so unwell, they had to stop the infusion. They still hadn't figured out I was allergic to a strand in the chemo. That's why I was so goddamn sick.

My oncologist made the call that I didn't have to finish the infusion, but that I would need to keep taking the oral chemo. I stayed in hospital overnight and got ready to leave the next morning.

The long, dark night

'I'm not taking the rest of my chemo tablets,' I told the nurses on my way out.

'You've still got two weeks left,' one of the nurses replied.

'I can't.'

A switch had been flipped. As soon as I said, 'I can't,' I was done. It's true what they say: the mind is a powerful tool. That works both ways. Your mind can get you through the hardest days, but it can also draw a line in the sand. I had hit a mental wall. Most people don't get to hit that wall because they're already dead.

Up until that point, my mentality had always been, if you can, you must. I no longer could.

I begged my oncologist for a break, for another option, for anything other than what I had been doing.

'If you stop now, you might need to do an extra six rounds of treatment,' the oncologist said.

'I couldn't finish the infusion. There's no way I'll be able to do another two weeks. These next two weeks of tablets are so minuscule compared to the rest of the regime. Are they really going to be the difference between the cancer being gone or not? You're going to remove whatever's left of the tumour anyway. Can't we do the surgery first and then see if I need more chemo? I need to do something else to keep moving forward. I can't keep doing this,' I reasoned. 'I know you're trying to save my life, but right now you're ruining it.'

'You've just got to do another two weeks,' he repeated.

'I can't do it. Why aren't you listening to me?' I cried. I yelled. I broke down.

'It's what's for the best,' he said, like a record player.

I asked Mum to leave the room—she didn't need to see this—and she went to get a Coke from the vending machine. I called nurse Emily, who was working in the hospital, and asked her to please come to the oncologist's office. She might have thought I was being a bit of a brat refusing to finish the next two weeks, but as soon as she walked into the office and saw me, she knew.

'She's done,' Emily told the oncologist, repeating what I'd already said. 'She's hit the wall. Look at her. Her body's done, her mind's done, she needs something new. Just tell her she doesn't have to do the next one.'

We'd reached a stalemate. It honestly felt like it was me (and Emily) against the world.

Jeremy was so worried about me. He pushed me to keep doing the chemo because that was what the doctors recommended. It was a black-and-white, logical, straightforward decision from where he was standing. But he wasn't the one sitting in the chemo chair. He didn't understand, and I couldn't find a way to explain it to him.

Emily organised an appointment with Dr G the next morning. It was decided that we'd pause chemo for the moment, and Dr G would go in and do a scope to see where

The long, dark night

things were at. I didn't know what would come from that, but I knew I couldn't finish my current regime.

I wasn't living, I was dying. The treatment was killing the cancer, but it was also killing me.

There must be another way, I thought. *There must be more.*

7
Silence as an act of survival

We didn't talk about the cancer at home. Or anywhere outside the hospital, actually. I didn't have the words—and even if I did, I wouldn't have known how to say them out loud. I was trying so hard to hold things together; I couldn't risk opening the floodgates. I knew I couldn't hack having a D&M with Jeremy or my mum. I didn't want to talk about my feelings; I wanted to get on with shit.

I had a therapist, but I didn't even speak to them about my fears or the reality of what I was going through. Mostly I just whinged about issues I was having with Jeremy. Looking back, a lot of those issues could've been avoided if we had better, more open communication, but that wasn't an option for me at the time. I couldn't lose focus by opening up about my emotions. I couldn't dwell on the fact that I'd spent most of my daughter's life in hospital. I couldn't wallow in thoughts about how my mum was being more of a mother to Sophia than I was. I couldn't do anything except what was necessary to stay alive. For Sophia.

We were all in survival mode. After Mum came to Adelaide when I was diagnosed, she never left. Mum had to leave Dad and my brother to fend for themselves in Port Lincoln, and she eventually had to give up her job and income to look after me and Sophia. I didn't know it then, but Mum thought I was going to die. It broke her heart to hear me crying at night, desperate to give Sophia her bottle and put her to bed, but unable to do so.

'I was absolutely gutted. I felt useless, hence why I came over [to live in Adelaide],' Mum said in an interview for the *Herald Sun*. 'They [Kellie and Jeremy] are both kids. They've never been through anything like this. They don't know how to process it. It's gut wrenching.'

Mum described our house as a war zone. 'They are young and they weren't expressing anything. Kell wasn't expressing how she was feeling. Jezz wasn't expressing how he was feeling, nor was I,' she said in the interview. 'We were bottling it up to keep the house happy. We didn't know how to talk. There was lots of bickering in the house. You'd say something and it would relay down to a fight with somebody.'

And so, silence became the default.

Another thing I didn't know at the time was that Jeremy was breaking down when he was on his own. He'd wait until he was alone in bed at night (in the spare room) or go out to the shed in the backyard. Like many blokes—my dad included, as I mentioned—Jeremy found solace in the shed. But, unlike most blokes, he wasn't doing the clichéd 'hiding from his wife's nagging'; he was hiding from my terminal illness.

'The shed was my place to escape and let it all out,' Jeremy said later. 'I was crying a lot behind closed doors. I didn't want Kell to see me. She was obviously gutted and upset, I didn't want to add to that.'

Jeremy also tried to keep it together at work. He knew he had a job to do there, and he was focused on providing for me and Soph. As much as he tried, though, it all spilled out one day at the club. Ash, the Port Adelaide physio, asked Jezz how he was doing. He started to answer, but only sobs came out.

Jezz was so embarrassed. Even though it's bullshit, there's still an unspoken rule that men shouldn't cry. Jezz asked the team's welfare manager, Paul, to send email updates to the team to stop people asking him how he was while he was at work. That helped Jezz to be able to go to work and keep a roof over our heads, without others' sad eyes reminding him that he had a sick wife at home.

Our approach to handling our emotions—burying them—wasn't healthy, but it was how we got through.

In June, we got news that Zac's sister was not doing well. While undergoing treatment for a second time, she lost all of her hair again and became more fragile than ever before.

Six months after finding out she'd relapsed, she was gone. The loss was devastating for everyone, especially those closest to her. We rallied around Zac and Rachel as best we could. My heart was with the family, but I must admit, a small part of it ached for myself, too.

The loss of Zac's sister was a reminder of what my reality could be; that I too could relapse, I too could leave my family behind.

Football was a much-needed outlet for Jeremy. If it wasn't for the game, he wouldn't have had any escape from the shit going on in our lives. Footy, the club and his fellow players kept him from spiralling. I was grateful he had the sport to lean on, because I certainly wasn't any help to him.

My sole focus was on getting through each day. Still, I tried to be as supportive as I could. After treatment, I would spend a week working hard to get better for Jeremy's game. If Jeremy was playing an away game, I would tune in from the couch. If he was playing on home turf at Adelaide Oval, I would do everything I could to be there and cheer him on with Soph. Watching him run out onto the field and play the game he loves was the only time I saw him truly happy during that period of our life. We owe a lot to AFL.

In spite of what was going on at home, Jeremy was giving it all on the field. Footy-wise, he was having the best year he'd ever had. He was channelling all the bullshit and putting it into his game. Jezz started wearing an armband on his wrist with my name written on it to remind him what he was playing for. He'd salute with that arm every time he scored a goal.

I'm always proud when he scores a goal, but honestly, I was most proud he was even able to strap up his boots and take to the field during that time. I don't think anyone would have blamed him if he decided to crumble and take some time out considering everything that was going on. But he powered through, and he did it for me and Sophia. Every time someone questioned his ability to show up, he would remind them that if I could show up and watch him at work and pretend life was okay for three hours a week, he could show up on the field. He supported me through his actions.

I would never have asked or expected Jeremy to take a break from football. He knew how much I loved watching him do what he does best, so he continued to do so to put a smile on my face.

~

I hadn't planned on falling in love. In fact, I'd committed to being free. It was the late 2010s, and I was in my travel era—and I had the tattoo to prove it. I was in Amsterdam, on a big European adventure, when I got my intentions inked.

'Flights not feelings' was my life motto. My mum was convinced that I'd find the love of my life overseas and never come home. But I was adamant: my time, energy and money would be spent on experiences, not boyfriends.

For my tattoo, I settled on a fine line paper aeroplane on my wrist. It said 'flights not feelings' without actually saying it. Very relevant.

After graduating university with my teaching degree—and ending my long-time relationship with Jed—I boarded a one-way flight in 2018, in time for Euro summer. I was meant to be 'solo travelling', but in my first eight weeks of gallivanting, I only spent three days on my own. I met old friends at various places on my travels and made new ones along the way. I vividly remember a warm day in June when I woke up in Switzerland, had lunch in Italy and sipped champagne in France later in the evening. It was 6 June, and therefore my half birthday, and the entire Contiki group I was with—as well as anyone we walked past throughout the day—celebrated like it was my actual birthday. I'm talking a cake with sparklers, 'Happy Birthday' being sung on repeat, and different celebratory shots at each bar all night long.

The next day sucked, but I'd felt like a half-birthday queen the night before, so it really didn't bother me.

Europe was a revelation. Everything was so close. In Australia, two hours wouldn't get me out of the same state, let alone to another country. I found it amazing that I could spend $30 and an hour on a flight and be in a different country. And so I did. I posed in front of the Eiffel Tower, rode around the cobblestone streets of Munich and sailed through Croatia on a yacht. I caught the travel bug. Bad.

I love being submerged in an entirely new culture and exploring entirely new cities. In Europe, that feeling was magnified by a thousand. There was so much at my fingertips. It was exhilarating. I felt a kick of adrenaline each time I looked up a flight on the Skyscanner website.

I had been living in and travelling across Europe for fifteen months when I cooked up a surprise plan. I knew I was heading home to Australia, but my family and friends thought I had taken on another year of work at an international school. Only a handful of people—just enough to help me get to and from airports—knew the truth. My contact on the ground in Melbourne was a boy I'd met in Budapest the summer prior, who'd moved to Victoria. He was my first port of call when I landed back in Australia in August 2019. He picked me up from the international airport and dropped me at the unit where my besties were living in Glen Iris.

I waited at my friends' front door in the Melbourne cold until one of them got home from work. Mads was my first victim. I scared the shit out of her and copped her car keys to the head. We knew Annabel and Charlotte would be home from work soon, so we went inside and hid my bags and myself in her room. I got to surprise Annabel, followed closely by Charlotte and our friend Holly who she had just picked up from the train station. 'I knew it!' Charlotte proclaimed.

She probably did know it; I had enquired about her weekend plans more times than someone who was on the other side of the world should.

We had the most magic weekend together, but because my family still had no idea I was in Australia, we had to lie low. I'd told Mum I was on a 'staff retreat' with the international school team to explain why I wouldn't be in touch with her or posting on social media. Everyone in Melbourne was in on it, and made sure I wasn't in any of their Instagram photos. I was determined to surprise the hell out of my parents.

First up, I made it to Adelaide and surprised a few more friends, including my cousin Tess and my best friend Kobi, who was in tears quicker than I was. (And she's usually the tough one!) Next, I flew home to Port Lincoln where my brother distracted Mum at the front of the electrical shop she worked at (she did the books), while I snuck in the back. Another amazing moment ensued.

It turns out I love making my life into a movie scene... Who knew I had a flair for dramatics?

I spent spring in my home town, before moving to Melbourne to live with my besties. I had taken the teaching position at Loreto by then, but figured it'd be a pit stop for me before I headed off on another overseas adventure. Then Jeremy Finlayson slid into my DMs.

Everything changed. Jezz—and his blue eyes—screwed up all my plans! Even though I was living in Melbourne, and he was based in Sydney playing for GWS, we managed to see each other every couple of weeks. I'd fly up to see him in Sydney, and he'd stop in to see me in Melbourne when he had a game in Victoria. We were back and forth and up in the air—physically, but not emotionally. Even though we were doing the long-distance thing, we both knew we were in it for the long haul. It was serious.

I messaged my mum to tell her the news: Kellie's solo travel era was over.

'Turns out I'm catching flights for feelings,' I wrote.

~

No one understood how I was feeling.

'I'm done. I can't do it,' I said to my family, the nurses and my oncologist. I said it over and over again, but I didn't feel like I was being heard.

After my blow-up with the oncologist following the failure of my fifth chemo infusion, I had my appointment with Dr G. He booked me in for a colonoscopy the following Wednesday. 'If we do the scope and I'm happy with the results, you won't have to do the next round of chemo,' he explained.

That was enough for me. I would've done anything to get out of going through the same type of chemo again. In saying that, I was still scared of having to do the bowel prep for the colonoscopy. The last time—when I ended up spewing and shitting myself on the shower floor—had traumatised me. Dr G insisted things would be different. I had a stoma this time around, he explained; the laxatives would be going into a bag, rather than fighting to get past the tumour in my bowel and being forced out the other end instead.

To put me at ease, Dr G offered for me to do the bowel prep in hospital. He was being kind, but firm, with me. It's exactly what I needed at the time. I needed him to be understanding, and I also needed him to lay down the law. I trusted him so much; whatever he said, went.

The scope was locked in and the appointment was a week away. I had an unexpected week off from being a cancer patient. I didn't know what to do with myself! It was pure bliss. We decided to get our kicks while we could and booked a last-minute trip to the Adelaide Hills. We went with friends: Port Adelaide player Sam Powell-Pepper, his partner, Brya Waghorn, and their little girl, Frankie, who was born seven months after Sophia. It was winter, so we rugged up and hit the wineries and a gin distillery. I even had a drink. We toasted to the possibility that I wouldn't have to do more chemo. Cheers to that.

For the first time since I was diagnosed, I felt like myself again. I knew I had needed a break, and I was right. The little trip away made a world of difference to me.

I'm sure it did the same for Jeremy and Sophia.

When I returned to hospital to start the bowel prep for my scope, I did so with renewed energy. Of course, it helped that going through the (laxative) motions was so much easier with a colostomy bag. The concoction was going through me, and I didn't even need to get up to go to the toilet. I could've slept through it! I made that joke to my stoma nurse, Paula, and she joked back, 'You're not getting a catheter, you lazy bitch.' Ha.

To get me through the night, they attached a drain to my bag and connected it to another two-litre bag. I downed the bowel prep formula and watched it flow out of me with ease. It was a breeze. I thanked my lucky stars for my stoma.

The next morning, I woke up prepped and ready to go. And starving. Dr G organised for me to be the first cab off the rank on his scope schedule for the day.

'Great. We just need to empty your bottom,' Paula told me.

'What!?' I asked. 'How do you do that? My bowels are asleep.'

'You've got two options,' Paula explained. 'We can do it the traditional way by giving you an enema through your anus, which might squirt out your stoma. Or we can put the enema down your stoma and let it come out the other way.'

I didn't like the idea of shit squirting out my stoma, so I went with option number two. In the bathroom, I took off my bag so Paula could see both the holes: the active hole for the output and an inactive hole, which was essentially just the bottom end of my bowel that was disconnected. The inactive hole allowed me to deviate my stool but also it was still there so it could be reattached later. Paula threaded a catheter down the inactive hole and squirted some liquid into it as a test.

'Did you feel that?' she asked.

'Nup.'

'Good, it's the right one.'

I sat on the toilet while Paula squirted enema into my inactive stoma hole, flushing out my other 'inactive hole'. It was the first time using my bum in over six months and it was the weirdest feeling ever. I swear it was like turning a tap on. The liquid poured out of me. The process didn't take long at all because the enema didn't have far to travel.

'You're clean!' Paula declared. 'Good to go.'

I was taken down to theatre and given some of the good stuff. Of course, the moment I was drugged up, the surgeon we all called Dr McDreamy walked by. 'Oh, you're so handsome,' I cooed, high as a kite. Smooth, Kellie, smooth.

As if that wasn't enough, Dr McDreamy was the one who checked on me when I woke up from the anaesthesia. This time I didn't just embarrass myself: I threw my nurse into it. 'Paula's so right,' I said, once again referencing his handsomeness. (Sorry Paula!)

For a second, I thought I was still a bit high when Dr G told me how the scope went. 'Once your bloods are good, girl, we can do this,' he said. I didn't need more chemo; I could go straight in for my big surgery to remove whatever might have been left of the cancer. The operation was called an ultra-low anterior resection, and it involved removing my rectum and sigmoid colon (the S-shaped part of the large intestine, which becomes the rectum), plus any of the affected lymph nodes. There were hundreds of the latter. The surgery would leave me with my inner and outer sphincter, which meant I would still have control over my bowels.

It might sound terrifying—and it was—but the surgery was also the best-case scenario for me. I felt like a crushing weight had been lifted off my back. The crushing weight was the chemo. Without the sickness and stress of my infusions weighing down on me, I could breathe again. It was such a relief.

I just needed my bloods to play sport for the surgery to go ahead. My white and red blood cells needed to be at a certain level for it to be safe enough for me to be under anaesthesia for such a long time. The surgery I was having was major, and my blood cells would play a key role in keeping me alive.

As it went, my blood cell numbers were shit. The last round of chemo I'd had—and abandoned part way through— had shot me. My immune system was non-existent, and my blood cells weren't building back up. I couldn't have surgery because the risk of infection was too great. My initial surgery date of 8 June 2022 had to be postponed. It was so frustrating.

After failing the initial blood test, I went back in the next day, and every day after, in the hope that my results would improve. They didn't. It was devastating not being able to have the surgery I knew I desperately needed. I felt like I'd worked so hard to get to this point—and nearly died in the process—and it still wasn't enough. *Will it ever be enough?* I thought to myself.

I know, in the scheme of things, this is so trivial, but one of the reasons I wanted to have the surgery as soon as possible was because we'd booked a holiday to Hawaii in November. I wanted my stoma reversal to be done before that, so I didn't have a colostomy bag on vacay. The reversal had to happen six weeks before I could travel, so I had to have it in September for things to go to plan. And the reversal couldn't happen until I was three months post-surgery, which meant the surgery had to be before July. I was cutting it fine.

Eventually, I was given a tentative surgery date of 18 June. The day before, Jeremy invited me to go for an afternoon walk and coffee at Henley Beach. It was a cold and cloudy day, so I rugged Sophia up. We didn't know what the next day would bring, but I had a hunch about what the beach stroll might bring. I'd seen a large transaction on our bank statement and knew Jeremy had taken my dad out for a beer the night beforehand. I'd done my nails just in case . . .

As we walked along the sand, I kept looking to see if I could spot a photographer. I'd told Jeremy the only request I had if he was ever going to propose was that a photographer was there to capture the moment. I wish I could say I wanted the photos purely as keepsakes for Soph, but the truth was, it was for entirely superficial reasons. I'd always wanted an engagement shoot; I wanted a beautiful image to announce the special news. I'm sure, deep down, I also wanted the photos for Jeremy to show Sophia when she got older as a reminder of her mum, if that was needed. No doubt I also had my looming surgery in the back of my mind, too. But I buried those motivations and focused on the other—less morbid—reason: Instagram.

Where is the photographer? That's what I was thinking when Jeremy dropped down on one knee.

Luckily for Jezz, the photographer was hiding behind the jetty and captured it all. We posed under the jetty with Sophia in her little pink tracksuit and beanie. I was smiling from ear to ear. We were engaged! I was going to get married, to be a bride, to be a wife.

Jeremy told me he wanted me to have something pretty to look at when I was in hospital recovering from the surgery. The surgery didn't go ahead the next day, but at least I had something shiny to distract myself.

It was Thursday a week later when my phone rang. Nurse Emily was calling to tell me about my latest blood test results. 'They're really fucking close,' she said. 'We can let you come in tomorrow to get you prepped and we'll put you on the Saturday surgery list.'

A Saturday appointment was unheard of. It was only because Dr G had a major surgery cancellation that he could fit me in. It felt too good to be true, so I tried not to get my hopes up.

I checked in to the hospital on Friday night to start prep for a Saturday morning surgery. Jeremy dropped me off. 'See you in a few days,' I said, not knowing how long I would be in ICU for. The hospital was a 40-minute drive from our house, and I felt guilty making Jezz drive back and forth so much. I would have preferred him to stay at home with Sophia than come all that way to visit for the sake of visiting, especially if I was out of it.

My surgery was meant to take four hours. They started to put me under and then sat me up to give me an epidural. I woke up eight hours later in the ICU. When Dr G opened me up, he discovered that all of my organs and lymph nodes were fused to my back because of the radiation I'd had. That would explain the lower back pain I'd been having... At the time, I chalked it up to me being horizontal in bed so much, but there was more going on inside me.

Later, Dr G explained that the operation had taken so long because they had to carefully remove everything that was attached to my back. There were two other surgeons in the theatre helping him.

I don't remember much from the days after the surgery. It was a struggle to open my eyes. It felt like my eyelids were tied down with heavy bricks. It wasn't a nice feeling. I'd woken up from other procedures feeling happily groggy. This wasn't like that. It was scary how drowsy I was. I have a vague memory of Jeremy visiting me and I know it was at night because he was going to get dinner on the way home. That's all I remember.

What's a hazy memory for me is something Jeremy will never be able to forget. Seeing me in ICU after the surgery shocked him to the core. I had a central venous catheter inserted into a vein in my neck, cannulas in both arms, an ECG monitor attached to my chest, cords everywhere and oxygen tubes up my nose. I was covered in blood from being cut open and had an enormous bandage around the wound. I was so weak; I couldn't even hold Jeremy's hand. He held onto mine instead and gave it a reassuring squeeze.

'My neck hurts,' I kept repeating. 'My neck. It hurts. My neck.'

Eventually, a nurse came and removed the tape that held the catheter in place at my neck and disconnected it from the ketamine it was pumping straight into my central line for pain relief. Any wonder I was as high as a kite. Ketamine is a serious painkiller.

The nurse counted to three and ripped the catheter out. They have to do it quickly, otherwise it could get stuck. They didn't know why I was experiencing pain in my neck—I had that many painkillers in my system I couldn't even feel the incision in my stomach—so they took the catheter out to be safe, in case it was the start of an infection.

Poor Jeremy was there for the whole thing. I can't even imagine how weird—and confronting—that would've been for him. He told me later that it was the first time he really thought I was going to die. *Fuck, she's on her death bed here*, he thought to himself.

While Jeremy was feeling the weight of the situation, I was feeling sweet fuck all. I was doing so well, in fact, I was transferred out of ICU to a room on the colorectal ward, Five North, the next day. 'Do you think you can get up to get into the new bed?' a nurse asked me.

'Absolutely not,' I said. My legs were still numb from the epidural.

They picked me up with the sheets underneath me and moved me into my new bed. Every movement hurt, but the pain didn't dampen my spirits. I was so proud to be leaving ICU earlier than expected. The surgery was over, I'd done it, and I was on the mend. Dr G was pleased with how the operation went and confident that he'd removed all the cancer. Things were looking brighter by the day.

Once I got to my new room, which had a view over the city and Glenelg Beach, the nurse explained how my fentanyl button worked. I could press it every five minutes for pain relief. 'Only press it if you need it,' the nurse told me.

For the first couple of hours, I felt relatively well and didn't have to press the button. I thought I was doing *so* good.

I bragged about it to my ICU nurse who visited me on her way out at the end of her shift. 'Oh yeah,' she said. 'We pumped you full of ket before we moved you, so that won't wear off for a couple more hours.' That put a pin in my bluster.

It wasn't long before I was tapping the fentanyl button like it was a 'press for champagne' lever at a trendy bar. The pain hit me with a vengeance. 'Is there any more pain relief I can take?' I asked.

'We really want your bowel to wake up,' the nurse told me.

'Can my bowel wake up another day?' I tried.

I was cracking jokes and feeling chuffed with myself in Five North. This is what I didn't realise: I was in a high-priority room right next to the nurses' station, where my nurse sat and monitored me when she wasn't attending to me in the room. I essentially needed 24-hour surveillance. My nurse only had two patients: me and the person in the room next door. In a standard situation, a nurse can look after up to seven patients at any given time. I didn't grasp how high-priority I was or how major the surgery had been. It helped that my recovery was virtually textbook: I didn't have any major complications or setbacks, which again lulled me into a false sense of security. I didn't fully understand that I could have taken a turn at any moment and ended up on the other end of the spectrum.

I was told I would be in hospital for weeks following the surgery. When I was admitted on the Friday, I started fasting ahead of the operation. Afterwards, I was on a strict diet of liquids, custard and jelly, and soft mush. I was *starving*. The pureed food wasn't cutting it for me. It was the same feeling you get when you eat an apple when you're hungry: it only makes the hunger pangs worse. After six days of custard, I was desperate for a proper meal. But I was far too scared to do anything that wasn't recommended by the doctors and nurses.

I was grateful for all the visitors I had, but I also felt an overwhelming sense of guilt about them being there. It was bad enough I was in hospital; I didn't want to drag my loved ones there, too. The thought of being a burden ruined me, so I didn't ask for support when I needed it.

As you can probably tell by this point, independence is a huge thing to me. It's always been my strong point and something I pride myself on. Having my independence completely stripped, in all of the worst ways, shattered my confidence. I had never experienced low self-worth before; I've always been a super-confident person.

Leanne, Brya's mum, came to visit me almost every day and brought baby Frankie with her when Sophia wasn't able to come in on that day. Franks is like my second baby; I almost feel like I had more of a 'first year of motherhood' experience with her than I did with Soph. Brya explained that she couldn't come herself. She just couldn't see me like that. It was fair enough. I understood it would hurt to see a friend in that shape.

I didn't really want anyone to see me anyway.

Until it happened to me, I had never thought about the guilt people with an illness or serious injury experience. I wasn't prepared for the people I loved to see me in an intense amount of pain. They suffered when I suffered. They struggled with not being able to do anything to help, not knowing the right words to say, not wanting to overstep, but also wanting to care for me. It was hard all round. They felt helpless and I felt like a burden.

When I was on my own, I was bored and lonely and low. Darkness crept in. Social media became a blessing and a curse. It was a way for me to share and connect, but it was also my constant reminder that life was still moving forward for everyone else while mine was at a standstill. I couldn't expect people to put their lives on hold for me, I didn't want that, but I also wished I didn't have to see all the things I was missing out on in high definition. I know, I know; no one was forcing me to log on, but it's a hazard of our generation.

While I was doomscrolling late at night, most people in the southern hemisphere were asleep. I was lucky my friends from Europe were awake and I was able to be distracted from my thoughts in those hours. Whether they'd admit it or not, the nurses didn't enjoy midnight D&Ms and my family members couldn't stay awake all night, either. You'd think the opioids would have helped me sleep—they certainly did make me drowsy—but my sleeps were more like little catnaps. I was like a newborn refusing sleep, but desperately craving it.

I spent too much time alone with my thoughts in the four walls of my hospital room. There were moments when I thought I'd never get home. Moments when I thought that I might have said my last goodbyes. Moments when I forced myself to stay awake because I thought I'd be more likely to speak to Soph again if I didn't close my eyes. Moments in the middle of a fever or new infection when I questioned how much more my body could take. I never once considered life being easier on the other side, but in those moments when I was struggling, I really wished I had someone there holding my hand, or chatting to me on FaceTime, or checking in with a message.

If I had more people visiting and calling, I would have had less time alone with my thoughts. It felt like I had a never-ending bank of hours where I was awake and alone every day. The visits I did get didn't scratch the sides. One of the hardest parts of the entire experience was the isolation. Imagine if I lacked confidence, too! It would have been even more crushing.

Looking back now, I know I would have benefited from a podcast such as *Sh!t Talkers* (which I would go on to launch), to hear from people in similar situations and know I wasn't the only one going through this nightmare. I also think I would have benefited from a counsellor at the hospital: a voice of reason to remind me I was where I needed to be. Logically, I knew I was in the best place I could be for my health status, but it was also the last place I wanted to be. If someone was there to reassure me and explain how important it was for me to heal in hospital, that would have helped.

It was hard on me, but I knew it was so much harder for my daughter. I spent twelve days in a row away from Sophia. In that time, I only saw her for a total of six hours. I know how important the first year of life is for a baby's development, and my baby was growing up without me. During Sophia's hospital visits, I noticed her becoming more distant. She stopped saying, 'Mummy, Mummy, Mummy.' She no longer 'needed' me. The realisation made my heart ache. As much as I knew Sophia was safe with Mum and Jeremy, my arms felt empty without her.

Those days on my own, far from my daughter, were some of the most difficult I've had. I longed to be home. And I prayed that Sophia wouldn't feel my absence any more than she had already.

8

Three words

A membership to the bowel cancer club is something I wouldn't wish on anyone. Unfortunately, the number of members is on the rise. Bowel cancer is Australia's second most common cause of cancer-related death. It is the leading killer cancer in 25- to 45-year-olds. I didn't know that statistic until I joined the club.

From the time of my diagnosis, I connected online with a woman named Rhiannon from Melbourne who was in a very similar situation to me. She also got her diagnosis after giving birth to her first daughter, Henny, who was a few months older than Sophia. The only difference between us was that Rhiannon started her treatment with the intravenous chemo first and then had the radiation, whereas I did it the opposite way. 'Oh, you have the easiest part to come,' I told Rhiannon when she started the radiotherapy part of her treatment.

I know, I know, it's crazy that I considered any part of the treatment as 'easy'. But that's what it was, in my case. During my five weeks of radiation, I had radiotherapy every weekday. But the worst part of that for me was the drive to the hospital. It was inconvenient because it was a 40-minute trip each way, and hard because I had terrible carsickness—not from the treatment, just from the drive.

Sure, the radiation gave me a bit of fatigue, but it was the driving that bothered me the most. The oral chemotherapy was also difficult, but it was far less toxic than the intravenous chemotherapy that sent me into shock. It was, in comparison, the 'easy' bit. For me.

It wasn't the same case for Rhiannon. Because she didn't have a stoma yet, she felt the full effects of the radiation that I basically breezed through. She experienced diarrhoea, acidic wee and bladder issues. Her arsehole was red raw. 'Oops, sorry.' I apologised for getting her hopes up.

Rhiannon was one of the few people who understood what I was going through, because she was going through it, too. I was so grateful to have her in my corner, and to be in hers.

Our ultra-low anterior resection surgeries happened two days apart. A week or so later, Rhiannon messaged me. 'I shat,' she wrote, proudly.

I was so happy for her! The first shit after surgery was a big deal. It meant things were waking up and working inside. Meanwhile, I was still waiting for any movement at the station; the station being my bowels. *It can't be much longer*, I thought to myself.

Two days later—nine days after my surgery—it finally happened. My bowels moved (into my stoma bag) and I took a step towards going home. I was so over being in hospital. I was ready to sleep in my own bed, without all the beeping, checking and chatter of the ward. Before that could happen, though, I had to wait for the test results of the biopsy they performed during the surgery.

I was struggling with my mental health more than I ever had. My mind was consumed by the four walls of my room. In the past, I had always had a strong mind, in the sense that I felt like I was in control of my thoughts most of the time. That control started to slip away from me. I was falling into depression and it was affecting my ability to stay positive as well as the way my body was healing.

Over the weekend, I had a 'cover' doctor (not Dr G) because they all took turns to be on call. I was desperate to convince the cover doctor to send me home. He appeared in my room for his check-in, and before I could even start negotiating my way out, he told me that he'd been on the phone to Dr G who had prepped him to say 'no' and convince me that I was where I needed to be at this stage of my recovery. By which he meant in hospital, on the colorectal ward, with my nurses.

I still pled my case, but unfortunately the pros of being in the hospital far outweighed the cons. The main con was that I couldn't stand being in hospital and it was bringing me down. As soon as I started to doubt my ability to get through another day, a new infection started to show itself and my recovery was extended. It happened like clockwork. It was a catch 22: I needed to get out to get better, but I couldn't get out until I was better.

Later that same day, at about 7.30 p.m., Dr G popped in. He'd snuck away from his daughter's eighteenth birthday celebration at a nearby pub to check in on me, and assure me he wasn't keeping me there just for the sake of it. He reminded me that because of my age I could in fact be his daughter, and that, if his daughter were in my position, he would want her here. He told me if I had managed to manipulate my way out of the hospital only for something to go wrong, he would be distraught and take it very personally.

He cared. A lot.

On my eleventh day in hospital I got an update from Rhiannon. The news was even more exciting than her shitting. 'I'm in remission,' she told me.

The joy and relief I felt for Rhiannon was beyond. I was so excited—for her and me both. Because our journeys had been so parallel, Rhiannon's news gave me hope for myself. If Rhi was in remission, surely I would be too. Rhiannon was my friend, my confidante and my hope.

~

Three words

One of my best friends in primary school was a boy named Shaun Pascoe. We had the same palm lines on our hands, and we thought that made us twins. It didn't matter to us that we were from different cultural backgrounds—Shaun was Aboriginal—we were certain we were related. Shaun called my mum 'Mumsie', and though we didn't hang out outside of school hours, when we were at school we were like two peas in a pod. People often joked that we were dating (yuck: boy germs), but we would just laugh it off and remind people that would be incest. Because we were siblings.

I was born to be a boy. Remember how my parents mistook a foot for a penis in one of the pregnancy scans? Well, they didn't let me being a girl get in the way of raising me like their son. I certainly wasn't a princess, at home or at school. I spent recess and lunch playing tag, footy and sometimes, if the boys let me bowl or bat, cricket, too. (Fielding was boring.)

Shaun was always by my side, and I was by his. I even joined him for the weekly Wednesday catch-up with Nunga group, our school's cultural club. Without intention, Shaun taught me parts of his culture in a way that I'd understand them: not by the book, not what is taught in history class, but real, raw, current practices. I probably didn't realise how significant that knowledge was to me until I met Jeremy, a Yorta Yorta man, and was able to relate to so much of his upbringing without knowing him at all—purely through what Shaun had taught me. What a gift it was to have grown up with Shaun.

I've always had tight-knit friends. I think there's truth in quality over quantity, especially in relationships. Just like with Jeremy, once I'm in, I'm in deep. If we're mates, we're solid. I'm still close with my high school girlfriend Charlotte, and I've been best friends with Kobi since we were four. When Zac got together with Rachel (the girl he was Christmas shopping for when I rang him to tell him I was pregnant), we instantly clicked. The same went for me and Sam Powell-Pepper's partner, Brya, who's become such a light in my life.

My friend Tina was one of the first people I told about my diagnosis. It was after 6 p.m. when I called her and her phone was on do not disturb. When I kept calling, she knew immediately something serious had happened. 'No one's calling me at that time unless it's an emergency,' she explained to me later, when I asked her what she remembered about the night I found out I had bowel cancer. 'You messaged and said, "Tina, I have cancer." And I thought, *surely not*. I met you at your house and still couldn't believe it was true. I think I almost disassociated from the facts. It was just so fucked and unfair and unfathomable. I remember thinking, *It's Kellie, though. She'll never* not *get through this*.'

It was friends like Tina who did get me through it. And it was my girls—Charlotte, Kobi, Rachel and Brya—who got me down the aisle on my wedding day. On the morning of the wedding, we got ready together in a hotel room in the city.

Three words

We had breakfast mimosas, and the hair and make-up artists worked their magic on us. My bridal party all wore the same colour, a silky champagne, and the flower girls were in the cutest little dresses. It was a traditional wedding morning in every way, except one: the bride was terminally ill.

No one spoke about me being unwell. My hairdresser didn't mention my hair falling out. The make-up artist didn't flinch when she dusted bronzer over the chemo port in my chest. My mum swore she was only crying happy tears.

~

I was so sure I was getting good news, I set up my phone facing my hospital bed to record the moment for posterity. All week I had been excitedly telling my family I was going to be getting my biopsy results soon. I was expecting the best. I imagined how it would feel to tell everyone that it was over, that I was cancer-free. I practised saying the words. They tasted sweet in my mouth.

I was waiting to hear three words from Dr G: 'You're in remission.'

Instead, I got six: 'We can't say you're cancer-free.'

I didn't hear what he said next. I was ugly crying too hard. It was devastating.

'You're not in remission,' Dr G said. 'Even though the scans were clear, and I *think* I got everything, there were microscopic cancer cells in some of your lymph nodes.'

It wasn't a matter of *if* the cancer came back, it was a matter of *when*.

'How the fuck am I going to tell my family this isn't over?' I asked, distraught.

My first thought was for my family. My second was for me.

'Does that mean I have to do more chemo?' I asked.

'No, there's nothing more you can do. Your scans are clear. But microscopic cells don't show up on scans. Even if you do have microscopic cells we can't see, we can't just keep killing you with chemo because of them,' Dr G explained. 'You're now completely stable. After your six weeks of surgery recovery, you can go and live your life.'

'Stable isn't remission,' I said.

It didn't make sense to me. Rhiannon—who had the same diagnosis and almost the same treatment as me—was in remission. Why wasn't I?

For eight months I had crawled through hell trying to get to the other side: remission. I made it to the gates, but they were locked. I didn't get to hear the words, 'You're in remission.' Instead of being 'cancer-free', I was 'stable'. It was cruel to be so close and yet feel so far away.

A quiet voice in my head questioned if things would have been different had I finished my final round of intravenous chemo. *What if, what if, what if?*

Dr G assured me that wasn't the case. 'There was nothing left for the chemo to attack,' he said.

Three words

The cancer was gone, but I wasn't free of it.

Instead of capturing happy news, my camera caught the moment my world shattered—again. I covered my face with my hands in disbelief and defeat.

Later that day, still numb with shock, I posted the video on Instagram. I'd been sharing little updates about my diagnosis on my account (mostly so I didn't have to call every person in my life), and I wanted to show the reality of what I was experiencing.

'Today I should be updating all my friends and family with the news that I'm in remission, that I had a complete response to the aggressive treatment and that my resection biopsy showed no remaining cancer, that I was going to be able to spend the rest of my life really living,' I wrote. 'Instead, today I'm sharing that my journey's not over, in fact it's only really just starting. There wasn't a complete response, and although my surgeon and team are genuinely stoked with the results considering the aggressive nature of the cancer I was diagnosed with, and there is a high chance that I am in fact going to be fine, it means the shadow of doubt and the unknown are still very much my reality.'

The response to the post was overwhelming. I had so much support from people I knew, as well as complete strangers. 'Sending lots of love your way,' people wrote. 'Stay strong and fight like hell,' they encouraged. 'You still got this,' they assured.

I was grateful for the kindness. And still numb from the news.

It wasn't over.

Worse still, I wasn't even allowed to go home and be with my family. Dr G told me I had to stay in hospital. I wrote a letter to him in my defence. 'I can't be in here anymore,' I said. 'If you want me to recover, you know I need people around me. I have to go home.'

The next morning, Dr G gave me a list of requirements. I had to keep my incision dressing clean. I had to come back to the hospital in two days to have it changed. And I had to see Paula at the same time to have my stoma checked.

I would've done anything to get home, so I made a pact with Dr G to follow his list. Even if I did spend the next six weeks in bed recovering, at least I could be in bed with Sophia. And an average-sized TV. And a fridge full of real food. And, oh yeah, my husband.

Home called.

~

I was a shell of myself. Worse than that, I was a potato lying in a bed. At my lowest, I got down to 42 kilograms. My average weight was 55 kilograms—and when I was pregnant with Sophia, I was 78 kilograms—so it was a significant difference. My body wasn't getting a lot of nutrients because

Three words

all the food I ate was coming straight out. Within twenty minutes of swallowing something, it would come out as a liquid in my bag. My body didn't have a chance to absorb any goodness.

Originally, I had a colostomy, but during my lower anterior surgery, I was given an ileostomy, meaning they attached my small intestine to my stoma, and what was left of my large bowel to my anus, so that my bowel was completely asleep.

I was severely underweight, but because everything was in proportion, I didn't look super unwell. I was skinny, but not disturbingly. I started taking a pure protein supplement to help me put on weight. It made me go to the toilet a lot—which didn't matter to me because I had a bag—but I got up to 48 kilograms. At that weight, I felt like I could walk without breaking.

I had decided that if I *looked* well, I would *be* well. I wanted to look like myself: Kellie. Not Kellie the Cancer Patient. I didn't want people to treat me differently, and I knew they would if I looked like I was sick.

I did my best to look 'normal', but that was sometimes a double-edged sword. When I was out in public, I had to carry all my stoma supplies with me and use the disabled toilet to change my bag. When I had Sophia with me, people probably thought I was carrying a baby bag. Little did they know I was cleaning up my own shit, not my daughter's.

Once, when I was out in public and had to change my colostomy bag, someone questioned me about being in the line for the disabled toilet. 'Uh, this is for disabled people,' they said.

'I know,' I replied, holding the bag I had to carry with all my colostomy supplies. 'Do you want to help me change my colostomy bag? I can't do it in a single toilet cubicle. I need a mirror.'

For so long, I had planned my life around my chemo sessions. If I had an infusion on a Wednesday, I knew I would be wrecked for the rest of the week. I would write off the weekend and hope to come good by the following Monday. On a well day, I could play with my daughter, go for a beach walk, grab a coffee and have an early dinner with Jeremy. On an unwell day, I prayed for time to go faster.

Now that I was without a treatment schedule dictating my days, I found myself a bit lost. Dr G had told me to go out and live my life, but that was easier said than done with a monstrous cloud hanging over my head.

We celebrated Sophia's first birthday with a sprinkle cake at home. Our little girl was growing up so fast. She was toddling around and saying more words than I expected a one year old to know. Her favourites were Mum, Dad, dog, no, nummy (dummy) and Lala. (Lala was her nickname for Frankie, because Sophia caught on to us calling her a sooky lala. Oops. They really are sponges.) Sophia loved the beach and the sun (just like her mum), and more than anything she loved breaking down for a boogie at any and every chance she got. Her hips have never lied.

'Happy birthday beautiful girl,' Jeremy wrote in an Instagram caption celebrating Soph's birthday. 'And well done Mum on a whole year of surviving motherhood and everything else.'

Jeremy had seen me at my best and worst in the first year of our daughter's life. There was certainly a sense of 'If we can get through this, we can get through anything.'

A week after Sophia's birthday, we flew to the Whitsundays for a family holiday in the warmth. I was determined to make Sophia's second year better than her first. Getting away was a good distraction, but I carried an uneasiness with me. It felt like something was caught in the back of my throat. And no matter how much water I drank or how hard I swallowed, it wouldn't budge.

I knew I had to learn to live with the knowledge that I wasn't cancer-free, but I didn't know how. If I wasn't doing treatment to fight the cancer, what was I doing? Waiting for the cancer to return with a vengeance? I don't have that kind of patience.

I filled up my days with other things. After the Whitsundays, I planned a little mum and bub vacay on the Gold Coast for me and Sophia while Jeremy was on an AFL trip to remote communities in the Anangu Pitjantjatjara Yankunytjatjara

Lands of the Northern Territory. I caught up with my friend Liv Cummings, who had given birth to her daughter, Halo, on the same day I had Sophia. It was so cute seeing the girls reunited; they were honestly like twins separated at birth.

After three months off the cancer hamster wheel, I had to return to hospital for my stoma reversal. The surgery attached my bowels back together in the hope they'd remember to function normally again. When I first had the colostomy, I hated my stoma. I couldn't look at myself fully in the mirror because of it. But as I went through treatment, I became more and more grateful for it, and the pain it saved me from. Still, I wasn't sad to see it go. I was ready.

But I wasn't entirely prepared to learn that for the 5-cent-piece-sized incision in my stomach to heal properly (and to avoid infection, given it had been a site through which I'd shat), it would be left open to heal on its own. I had a wound that looked like a gunshot on my stomach. It was almost harder to look at than the stoma itself.

In the hospital after the reversal, I was starving. The custard and mushy veggies weren't cutting it for me. I was cheeky and ordered mac and cheese online and got one of my friends, Kiera, who happened to be a nurse in the hospital I was in, to sneak it in for me. She became a frequent flyer in my room: before work, during lunch and dinner breaks and on her way out when her shifts ended. She was always keeping an eye on me, always making sure I was taken care of.

Three words

One extremely busy morning on the ward, Kiera was clocking off from a night shift and I was yet to be tended to, so she took it upon herself to get my morning meds sorted. Hell, she even changed my wound dressing for me. Now, *that* is true love.

Once I was able to, I spent hours every day doing 'hot laps' around the ward. Five North became my runway and the nurses began anticipating my strut. I walked past them at least three times a day, trying to get things moving inside me. At the time, my friend Jordy, who has severe Crohn's disease, was in the room opposite me. She'd just got her first stoma after twenty-something years of living with the disease, and she became my hot lap buddy.

I took the hot laps very seriously.

~

I've always been competitive. From the little girl playing AFL against the boys to the adult on the netball court, I love to win. And I'm a pretty shit loser.

That was never more obvious than during an exercise physiology class at university. We were playing a game of indoor footy and I was pitted against a bloke on the opposite team who must have been 195 centimetres tall. No doubt he thought he had me beat. Little did he know.

We dove for the ball at the same time and I gave my leap everything I had. I landed on top of the ball and my opposition landed on me. When I stood up—victoriously—I was expecting cheers, but I only got shocked stares.

'Tooth!' someone said.

I reached for my mouth, but my teeth were fine.

'Not yours. His.'

That's when I noticed the stinging feeling, and the blood pouring out of my head. My opponent had landed on me with his mouth open and his front tooth was lodged in my forehead. It had snapped straight off from his gum. The big bloke came over to me and casually picked his tooth out of my head. There was so much blood.

My fellow students rallied to find a first-aid kit, rinsed the wound out with saline and wrapped my head with gauze. Someone drove me to a nearby hospital where they stitched me up.

I still have a scar today, but the guy got off much worse. They managed to glue his tooth back in, but he was never able to eat an apple again. Poor fella. And he had to live with the knowledge that I beat him to the ball. I won. In all the drama and blood, that point may have been overlooked, so I'm reminding everyone here. Victory sure is sweet.

~

Our hospital hot laps looked something like this: two tiny little brunette girls (malnutrition was evident in

Three words

our appearance), in matching pink silk Peter Alexander pyjamas and fluffy slippers, with large hot coffees in our hands, walking at a slow but impressive pace around the ward. Nurse Paula spent 90 per cent of her shift between our rooms. I don't know if that was because we were her favourites, or her most troublesome. Regardless, I was less lonely with her around.

While I was trying to get my bowels moving, Jordy had the opposite problem. Her bowels were moving too much, and what was coming out was acidic, and painful because it was so constant. I felt for her, and she felt for me. I thanked my lucky stars for the stoma that I had once more when I saw Jordy's. The skin around her stoma looked as though it was being eaten away. It looked so sore, and I know it was. Jordy and I understood each other on a deeper level. We bonded over our bowels.

Within a week of being home after my reversal, I asked Paula, 'How hard is it to put the stoma back on?' I realised more than ever how much it had saved me.

I had to learn how to shit again. Being incontinent as an adult—especially as an adult with a baby—is wild. I was changing my nappies after changing Sophia's. I'll never forget the moment I shat myself in Jeremy's car, with Sophia in the back seat. We were driving home from the hospital after a scope, so I had laxatives in my system. I suddenly felt an almighty cramp. 'I've got to go, I've got to go!' I told Jezz, sitting on the edge of the front passenger seat. 'I can't hold it in anymore. It's coming. It's coming.'

I desperately grabbed a nappy from Sophia's nappy bag and put it between my legs. I didn't know what else to do. What came out of me was disgusting. It stank like nothing I've ever smelled before. When Jeremy pulled over on the side of the road, I hopped out and stood there, naked from the waist down, with a kid's nappy between my legs. It was a Sunday afternoon, so the road was quiet at least—or so I thought. Then I saw a person walking their dog on a leisurely weekend stroll. *Fuck me*, I thought. *That poor woman. She'll never be able to unsee this.*

I fastened the nappy around me and put a second one down on the front seat. 'Go, go, go!' I told Jeremy. 'Get me home to a toilet.'

As soon as we pulled up, I ran inside clutching my nappies. Of course, our neighbours were out the front of their house, and saw me in all my glory.

It was traumatising in the moment, but as soon as we got home and I sat on the toilet, we started howling with laughter. I was afraid to move from the toilet, not knowing what else might come out, so Jeremy came and sat on the bathroom floor with Sophia. We were laughing hysterically. Soph was so confused. She'd never seen us act like that. She must have thought we'd lost the plot. Maybe we had.

It took me a while to get used to not having a rectum. Because I still had my sphincter, I had some control over my

Three words

bowels, but I didn't know whether a fart was going to be a wet one. Jeremy would joke while he was putting the laundry in the washing machine. 'One pair of knickers, two pairs of knickers,' he'd tease. 'How many is that this week?'

We laughed about it because that's all we could do. Everyone shits. It's human and natural. But talking about poo with your partner isn't romantic. Laughing through it was the only way. If you don't laugh . . .

9
The true cost

I made a living list. The thought of a bucket list—things to do before you kick the bucket—was too morbid for me. I didn't want to count down the days until I died; I wanted to cherish my time alive.

There were some big goals at the top of the list: to get married, buy a home and go on an African safari. I was shooting for the stars. The list also included some simple items: to take Sophia to her first dance class, to teach her how to swim, and to see her start daycare. But, first things first: we were going to Hawaii.

While I was waiting for my major surgery to be scheduled, the thought that kept me going was of sinking my toes into the sand of a Hawaiian beach. We didn't know if it would be possible. I needed six weeks to recover from my stoma reversal before I could travel. The reversal had happened in the nick of time, and I was giddy with glee boarding the flight to paradise.

By the time we landed in Honolulu, I hadn't slept for 48 hours because of the travel—but it didn't matter. I was in Hawaii with my fiancé and my baby girl. Sophia was in her element. Her hair was just long enough to put in a little ponytail on the top of her head, and she had a suitcase full of adorable floral holiday outfits. We had twelve days on the island of Oahu. We hired a car so we could explore.

It wasn't long before we slipped into a holiday routine. The mornings were usually slow: a stroll down the main strip to the cafe on the beach where the staff knew our order in just a few days. Soph was bringing main-character energy and everyone, including myself and Jezz, would watch her dance and play all morning until it was time for her midday nap. Jezz would join her, which meant: *me time*. What a treat! Some days I would spend time at the lagoon or by the pool with a book, or even on a sneaky trip to the shops. It was the first and probably last family holiday that had an element of relaxing (because Sophia no longer naps).

We did a lot of scenic hikes, but one stands out in my mind. I'm not sure why; there's no particular reason. We just happened to be interrupted by Jason Momoa filming his upcoming TV series *Chief of War*, with nothing but a rag wrapped around his waist.

The true cost

The sight made me forget my own reality. And I welcomed the distraction.

We had originally planned to see more of the US while we were in Hawaii, but because of my health, and the limited time we had before Jeremy started his preseason training, we stuck to Hawaii. Don't get me wrong; I'm not complaining! I was grateful to be having a holiday at all. I had been dreaming of it for so long.

As great as it was, the holiday was a reminder of all the things I'd sacrificed in the last year, and all the things I would need to sacrifice in the future. Travel has always been such an important part of my life, and I vowed to prioritise it where I could. It all came back to my quality of life. In the trenches of treatment, I asked myself, *What is the point of being alive if I'm not really living?* And the same sentiment remained.

Tomorrow isn't guaranteed. Today is a gift.

~

It wasn't culture shock so much as culture awe. *Holy shit, everyone is so happy here!* I thought to myself when I touched down in Norway. I'd grown up hearing stories of Norway from my mum, who lived there with her adoptive parents when she was a teenager. I had always wanted to visit the place where my maternal grandfather was from and where my mum called home. In Australia, Mum's name is Jane Marie; in Norway, it's pronounced 'Yana Maria', which sounds so much more exciting and exotic.

Some of my cousins had travelled to Norway when they turned eighteen, and I was so envious of them. I finally got the opportunity when I went travelling in 2018. The plan was to land in Norway, spend a couple of weeks with my family there, and then travel through Europe, doing a Contiki tour and a Sail Croatia cruise, and hopefully a stint nannying in London. I'd had a couple of phone interviews with families before I left Australia.

I had it all worked out. But the universe had other plans for me.

I was staying with my mum's cousins in the town of Arendal, the place I'd heard stories about as a kid. It was exactly like something out of a storybook, too. There were pastel-coloured buildings, a postcard-worthy harbour and cobblestone laneways. It's the place that inspired the town Arendelle in *Frozen*. I walked around in a state of amazement.

But I soon learned not to gawk like a tourist, because Norwegians hate tourists. People in Norway don't smile or say g'day to strangers on the street. It's an introverted country. The only time someone said hello to me was when I passed them on a hike. Norwegians are not rude, they just don't suffer fools or tourists. I swear the Norwegian prices are so high on purpose, so no one else can afford to visit.

The true cost

I tried to live like a local during my couple of weeks there. I took public transport to get around, spoke broken Norwegian, visited my family's ski cabin and hung out with my cousins. I got to see the home where my mum had grown up, which was such a full-circle moment. I didn't realise how much it would mean to me until I was there. I took a photo in the same spot where my mum and her siblings posed for a picture at the start of each school year. It was wild to me: to be walking a path my mum had walked before me, on the other side of the world.

My mum has never drunk coffee, because she was scared off it by Norwegian coffee when she was younger. It's not like the flat whites or long blacks we have in Australia; it's more like a bitter cold brew. Norwegians put a sugar cube on their tongue before they drink it—probably to make it palatable. I set out to find a decent cuppa in Arendal and found Unwrapped. It was eco-friendly—people brought their own containers for takeaway orders—and it was the only place that had alternative milks. At the time, I thought I was lactose intolerant because of my infrequent bowel movements, so I wasn't drinking dairy milk. The cafe was run by an American, who happened to be the wife of the principal at the local international school. I spent so much time at the cafe I got to know the owner quite well—so much so, she went home and told her husband all about me: the qualified teacher from Australia with roots in Arendal, hoping to stay and work in Europe.

Can you see where this is going? The principal asked me to come in for an interview. When we realised my cousins had gone to the school when they were younger, it felt like a sign. I was offered a teacher's aide position, with a nine-day fortnight and the same salary as a teacher. It was a dream come true, with one single downside: the job started a week before I was due to finish my European adventure, so I had to cut my holiday short. That and my flight from Portugal back to Norway was astronomical because it was peak season, and I was booking last minute. I reminded myself I was spending money to make money.

I went to the police station to apply for a residency visa, which was fast-tracked because my mum had a Norwegian passport and my aunty came with me. The authorities approved the paperwork and the school sent me a contract. I was in a hostel in London, the night before the start of my Contiki tour, when I had a video call meeting with my new employers to finalise the details.

When I returned to Norway after my Euro summer adventure, it was as a resident. My aunty—bless her—had organised a rental for me. It was a little one-bedroom cabin with a quaint living and dining room. The accommodation was called Home of Vench and Bjorn (the names of the owners), but in English it translated to Home of Wench and Bjorn, which was really fun to write on forms. The cabin had everything I needed, and was walking distance to a grocer,

The true cost

the bus stop and town. Best of all, it was 500 metres from the school I'd be working at.

I had a home group class of fifteen kids in Grade 7. Because it was an international school, the kids spoke more English than Norwegian. They only really spoke in Norwegian when they didn't want me to understand—little did they know I had learned all the swear words. I didn't need to use my secret talent much; the kids were so beautiful and polite. God they were good kids.

In Norway, the teacher–student bond is close. The kids became almost like family to me, which might sound weird, but that's how it is over there. The AFL Grand Final was airing on the last day of school before a break. My team was playing, so I taught my class the Collingwood song. We watched the game and they sang the Magpies anthem with me in solidarity. It didn't help; we still lost. The next day I got so many emails from the kids rubbing it in, knowing I wouldn't see them for the next couple of weeks on term break to tell them off.

The first day it snowed, my Grade 9s called me outside to see how beautiful it was. They were right: it was breathtaking. I was admiring the magnificence when the first snowball hit. The kids had lured me outside to attack me with snow. I was the only teacher they could go absolutely all out on without getting in trouble; they knew I was loving it almost as much as they were.

There Must Be More

I made friends with the two other expat teachers who started at the school the same year as me: Lorelei and Cindy. We started going to the gym together most mornings and doing a Zumba class every Friday night. We'd go for dinner afterwards and be in bed by 7 p.m. Everything happened early in Norway: we rose early and rested early. The slow pace felt good.

∼

When we returned to Adelaide from Hawaii, I got to cross another item off my living list. I took my baby girl to her first day of daycare. Sophia was so much more ready than I was. She wore an adorable pair of pink overalls, a backpack as big as she was, and her hair in tiny pigtails. She clapped her hands in excitement in the car on the way there. At daycare, she dug in the sandpit, played the rattle during music time and made new friends.

It was such a bittersweet moment for me. Of course, I was so happy to see her thrive, but I was also gutted at how quick the time had gone. My baby girl was all grown up. When did that happen?

To start with, Sophia only went to daycare one day a week. My mum had gone back to Port Lincoln after living with us for a year, and it was a huge adjustment for all of us. It must have been wild for Mum; she'd basically raised Soph for the first year of her life. I was worried Mum would have withdrawals.

I remember the moment realisation dawned on Mum as she was packing to go home. 'Fuck, I'm not going to see Sophia for three weeks,' she said. It was almost as though she was taken aback by the thought, as though it had hit her in the gut. It hurt. Mum had been with Soph every day since I was diagnosed. If Soph woke up at night when Jeremy was away and I was unwell, it was Mum who would settle her. Mum was basically the main carer. It wasn't a job she signed up for, but it was one she did with unconditional love. She didn't complain once.

I don't think I'll ever be able to thank my mum enough for everything she did for me, for us. She got hit the hardest with looking after us all, but she was the bravest.

As excited as I was to get into our own routine as a family of three, I knew I would miss Mum, too. I was also a little bit scared to be taking on everything on my own. I wasn't used to it.

Luckily, Mum got a job with a company based in Adelaide, so she would spend a couple of days a week working in the office and staying with us. Often, she'd stay for the weekend to give me and Jeremy a hand and some quality time to ourselves if we needed it. (That's how she spun it to us, but we all know the quality time was for her and Soph. Ha.)

With Sophia in daycare and some extra time on my hands, I began to think about my own career. I hadn't taught since a few months before having Soph, and I was raring to get back to it. I started telling people I'd be back in the classroom in January. I was hoping to return to relief teaching instead of a full-time position, to ease back into it. I missed teaching so much. I get so much satisfaction when a kid 'gets' it, when everything clicks into place and they understand a concept or equation. It's such a fulfilling job.

In the meantime, I had some other unexpected work opportunities. I had signed with a management company earlier in the year—no doubt thanks to Jeremy being a footballer—and had a growing profile. After I posted the footage of myself reacting to the news I wasn't in remission, the video went viral. It got thousands of views and was picked up by different media outlets. I was officially given the title of 'Jeremy Finlayson's terminally ill wife', and I got more interest from brands in doing collabs. I was invited on Steph Claire Smith and Laura Henshaw's podcast, *KICPOD*, and *Life Uncut* with Brittany Hockley and Laura Byrne. I was interviewed for *The Project*, photographed on red carpets and being styled for events by my now good friend Lauren Dilena.

It was satisfying to be working in whatever form that took. For an entire year, my career had been on pause. There were plenty of moments when I felt like I was being left behind, stuck, at a forced stop. The world kept moving, but I was frozen in time. It felt daunting.

The true cost

I was ridiculously lucky to have private health insurance (thanks again, Mum), but the cost of having cancer still added up. As well as losing my income, Mum lost hers, too, when she quit her job to become my and Sophia's carer. We briefly looked into applying for a carer's allowance, but we didn't qualify for that because of Jeremy's salary. Mum was told to ask Jeremy for a wage if she couldn't afford to live off her savings. 'My son-in-law has just been told his partner is dying, he has a newborn baby and has just started a new job. I will not be asking him for money,' she replied.

It's expensive work being sick. I remember getting a bill in the mail for a surgery that cost $101,000. That one was covered by my insurance, but not all of them were. We were spending thousands of dollars a month on my health care. Anything that was handed to me as a prescription was an out-of-pocket expense. Oral chemotherapy? Yep, I had to pay for that, as well as the opioids, nausea and gastro medication, and scans. We spent literally thousands of dollars on scans every two to three months. Alternative therapies were not covered by my insurance, either. We made it work—and I guess that makes us privileged—but we didn't have any choice about it.

I distinctly remember the first time someone called me 'privileged sick'. It stung. The person was insinuating that my husband's job—and salary—made having cancer easier. Let me tell you, there's nothing easy about cancer. I understand that having private health insurance and being able to afford health care is a privilege, but being sick is not.

As the 2022 Christmas season approached it felt entirely different to the year before, when I'd been in the thick blur of diagnosis and treatment. It was going to be Sophia's second Christmas, and she was so much more aware of what was going on, which made things even more exciting. We put up a Christmas tree in our living room and decorated it with lights and baubles. Soph helped us put the star on top. I was determined to give her some happy Christmas memories to make up for the ones I missed the previous year. You better believe I was going to soak up all the summer sun I missed out on, too.

We headed to Port Lincoln to spend the holidays with my family and at the beach. It was all I ever wanted: sun, surf and Sophia. I was ready. I was excited. I was breathless . . .

Why the fuck was I breathless?

~

There's something truly magical about a white Christmas. It feels like the way Christmas should be (according to the movies anyway). The snow! The roast turkey! The ugly sweaters!

My Christmas in Norway was a world away from the cold prawns and beers of Chrissy in Australia, but a piece of Australia came to visit me on the other side of the world.

The true cost

My mum and brother came to Europe for the festive season. Dad hates flying—especially long haul in economy—so he stayed home, which was fair enough.

Jake had just turned eighteen, and we spent New Year's Eve in Amsterdam. Can you imagine how much fun we had? So much. My brother threw caution to the wind and had a ball. I was more sensible—I'd already spent six months in Europe and was a careful traveller—and yet I was still the one who got robbed. I don't know where or when it happened, but someone stole my wallet, phone and residency card. I went to pay for something in a store and realised my bag was gone. The thief had cut it from my body, and I hadn't even realised until that moment. Fuck.

Losing my money and phone was annoying, but those things could be replaced. My residency card wasn't as simple. I went to the Norwegian embassy in a panic and got a note from them to give to the authorities at the airport. When I got to the Norwegian security gates—carrying my note like a naughty little kid—my residency card was there. Someone had handed it in.

Merry Christmas to me.

~

I thought I had Covid. *Just my luck to get sick before Christmas*, I thought, shaking my head.

I went to the doctor in Port Lincoln to do a test, and luckily the nurse there knew me. She knew about my story and my bowel cancer. She set up a CT scan to be safe. Thank god she did. The scan showed a large mass in my chest cavity. The doctors weren't too worried, though, because they thought it was just pneumonia. All my symptoms suggested as much. They recommended I stay in Port Lincoln and enjoy the rest of my summer holiday there, before seeing a lung specialist when I got back to Adelaide in the new year.

Back in Adelaide, I was scheduled for a bronchoscopy. I sat across from the surgeon and levelled with him: it wasn't my first rodeo. 'Please, whatever happens, when I wake up, don't bullshit me. Tell me everything you can,' I said, before the anaesthesia took me to the land of dreams.

During the bronchoscopy, the surgeon discovered I had a collapsed lung. That explained my shortness of breath. He also found an artery that looked like it was clogged with mucus. The surgeon was cheering because he thought he could suck the mucus plug right out, and then I would heal up nicely. But when he did and it started bleeding, he knew he'd made a mistake. The mass was cancerous.

I had relapsed. My cancer was back. And it was in my lungs.

To see just how far it had spread I was booked for a PET scan. The process of a PET scan involves fasting before having a radioactive liquid infused with saline injected into your

The true cost

body. You have to sit still for an hour, while the infusion spreads, before lying in the machine that takes the scan. You have to be totally still for 30 minutes, and you can't fall asleep in case you twitch. It's like torture, especially when you're tired and hungry from fasting.

Because the cancer doesn't have any carbs or sugars to feed on, it sticks to the radioactive solution and, if its active, it glows on the PET scan. The scan picks up the tiniest traces of cancer and highlights them like a Staedtler marker.

I had to wait two days for my results. I went to see the lung doctor, who hadn't had a chance to look at my file before the appointment. I sat down in his office with Jeremy beside me. When the doctor turned the screen around to show me the PET scan results, I stood straight back up. 'No worries, thank you,' I said as I walked out the door.

I tapped my card and paid $1200 on the way out of the office. It was the most expensive two minutes of my life.

'Why did you walk out like that?' Jeremy was confused.

I didn't need to hear what the lung doctor had to say. The PET scan told me enough. There were highlights all over the screen. I knew the lung doctor wouldn't be able to operate, so there was no point being in his office.

The cancer was *everywhere*. It was all through my stomach, pelvis and lungs. I was riddled with it.

I sobbed with anger on the drive home. Raging, white-hot tears of fury.

10

Voice of reason

The advice was to 'go home and get comfortable'.

I had been given three options by my oncologist before I got the results of my PET scan in January 2023. If the cancer was just in my lung, the oncologist told me, they would operate and remove the cancer. If it was in my lung and the surrounding lymph nodes attached to the lung, they would remove the cancer and give me chemo to kill off any microscopic traces. If it had moved further than the lymph nodes attached to my lung, they would be looking at putting me in palliative care.

As soon as I saw the PET scan on the lung doctor's screen, I knew I was looking at the third—and worst—option on a dismal list. In the car on the way home, Jeremy didn't understand why I was so upset. I tried to explain what the oncologist had told me, but Jeremy didn't know what palliative care meant.

So there I was, sitting in the car on the way to pick up our one-year-old daughter from Brya and Sam's house, shuddering with sobs, trying to tell my fiancé that palliative care was the end of the road. It was game over. Do not pass go, do not collect $200.

'It means I go home, get comfortable and wait to die,' I said, trying to be gentle. But there was nothing gentle about what I was looking at down the barrel.

'What do you mean?' Jeremy kept asking. 'What do you mean? That can't be right. There must be another option.'

Of course I was going to get a second opinion. As defeated as I felt in the moment, I wasn't going to take my relapse lying down. I just needed to have a little cry first.

When we pulled up at Brya and Sam's place, Jeremy went inside to pick up Sophia who had been playing happily with Frankie. He didn't come back out for what felt like hours. I knew he would have been updating them, and also hopefully processing the news.

While he did that, I sat in the car and called nurse Emily and told her about the PET scan. Dr G called me straight back. He'd seen the scan. He could hear the urgency in my voice. He knew what it all meant.

'I need another opinion,' I said.

'Of course you do,' Dr G replied. ('No fucking shit,' is what I heard.)

Voice of reason

If it's not entirely obvious already, I didn't see eye to eye with my oncologist. I felt like he didn't hear me, and he certainly didn't understand me. Unlike Dr G and my nurses, the oncologist didn't get how important my quality of life was to my treatment. I needed a reason to live, to keep fighting to live. Dr G recognised how much stronger I was when I had people around me. He knew I healed better at home than in the hospital. He took note of what I needed, and he factored those things into my care.

My oncologist, on the other hand, didn't seem to give a shit. It was his way or the highway. I didn't have a say. My voice didn't matter. He made that clear when I was begging him to stop the intravenous chemo he'd prescribed—the one with a strand he didn't realise I was allergic to—and he told me I had to. I didn't have a choice.

So, when the oncologist offered up palliative care as my only option, I knew I needed to speak with another oncologist. I *was* going to have a choice.

During my first dance with the devil that is cancer, I followed my doctors' lead almost blindly. I didn't do my own research or seek out more information. I did as I was told. It felt like I was walking around in a haze. Everything was blurry—I couldn't see further than the step directly in front of me. No doubt I was experiencing some kind of shock.

This time around, the shock had worn off slightly. I had a better idea of what I was in for, and I was determined to do the work. I was going to be proactive, to ask the hard questions and to advocate for myself.

~

My first boss was a creep. He ran the shopping-centre bakery I worked at in high school, along with two of my friends, Caitlin and Charlotte. We were a close little trio. The shifts when we were rostered on together were the best because we had a laugh, and had each other's backs. We needed to. There was safety in numbers.

In the early days of working there, we used to fight to avoid the Sunday morning shift. None of us wanted to wake up early after a Saturday night. But as we got closer to finishing school, we used to fight to *get* the Sunday morning shift, because we were saving to go away for schoolies week and wanted the higher penalty rates.

As teenage girls, we weren't taught to stand up for ourselves. We were taught to be polite, to do as we were told, to smile because we look prettier like that. My friends and I weren't in a position to call out our boss's crappy jokes. We sucked it up. We figured it was just part of the job.

We might not have spoken up, but we got our revenge in a different way.

When we neared graduation, we all applied for leave to attend schoolies week. But the boss refused to give us time off.

'If you go to schoolies, don't come back,' he said.

And that's exactly what we did. We went away to Victor Harbor to celebrate with our mates, using the money we made on those Sunday shifts. We didn't go back, and the baker lost three employees in one fell swoop.

~

Jeremy didn't say anything at the time. A year passed before I found out what was going through his mind when I had to explain palliative care to him. That moment, Jeremy later explained, was the first in which he saw his life without me. He saw Sophia without her mum. He saw him as a single parent. That's all he could think of.

'I didn't even make it down Brya and Sam's hallway before I started bawling my eyes out,' Jeremy told me. 'I said, "She's got it again. It's all through her. This could be it." I couldn't stop crying.'

Brya remembers the same: Jeremy collapsed in tears. 'He literally fell into our arms in absolute tears as soon as he walked in,' she said. I guess that explains why he took so long to emerge from their house with Sophia.

Jeremy had been confronted with my mortality before—when I was in ICU after my major surgery, and he thought I was on my death bed—but he hadn't pictured his life without me. This was the first time he was facing the reality of losing me. I'd already faced it—that night in bed after my first round of intravenous chemo when I was sure I would die—and it was brutal.

As was the status quo with us, Jeremy didn't voice his fears with me. In fact, when he got back in the car—after venting to Brya and Sam—he seemed calmer. I'm sure he wasn't calm on the inside, but he held it together for me. I gave myself permission to fall apart for a moment, and then I pulled myself together, too.

The next day, I went to David Jones to get Sophia some new shoes for daycare because she inherited her feet from her dad, and they grow faster than weeds. I had shared an update on my health on Instagram, and the news had spread, again like a fast-growing weed. The local newspapers were still referring to me as 'Jeremy Finlayson's terminally ill wife', as though my marital status and my sickness were the most important things about me.

It was while I was browsing the kids' section at David Jones that it happened. A woman on the other side of a clothes rack stopped me. 'You look awfully well for someone who's terminally ill,' she said without hesitation.

Her tone suggested that I was lying about the extent of my disease, or that she didn't believe someone with a terminal illness could do ordinary things such as shop for their kid's shoes. Regardless, I was taken aback by the comment. From a stranger. In a department store. Sure, I'd gotten negative comments and DMs on social media before, but I didn't give them any air. It's one thing to receive anonymous messages on a screen, and another to face them in person. I didn't know how to respond to the woman. I walked out of the store empty-handed and paced my way back to the car. I called Brya's mum, Leanne, in a bit of a daze. I told her what had happened and she couldn't believe it, either.

I had to shake the shock off, though, because I had shit to do. I booked an appointment to meet with a new oncologist. I went in with Leanne as backup, and I was determined to speak up for myself and be heard. I was expecting war, because every interaction with my last oncologist had been a battle.

When I sat down with Dr T, I voiced my priorities. Of course, number one on that list was to stay alive, but I also explained that in order for me to do that, I needed to have a decent quality of life.

'I understand,' the doctor replied.

Um, sorry, what? I thought to myself. *Is this doctor actually listening to me?*

'So, what can we do differently to make treatment better for you?' the doctor asked. 'What didn't work last time? What do you need more of this time?'

They were the exact questions I needed to be asked. I answered honestly—I *really* didn't want to do chemo—and the doctor replied in kind.

'I'm sorry, but chemotherapy is your only option,' he levelled with me. 'We can do targeted radiotherapy and other things, but chemo is the best option for you. You're riddled with cancer and we need to mop that up before we can do anything else.'

'Alright, I can do it. I don't want to do it, but I can,' I relented.

'Good. We can't put you on the same chemo as last time, though, so we'll put you on another type. The side effects won't be as severe,' he explained, giving me the good news first. The bad quickly followed: 'You're going to lose your hair, and you'll need to have a chemo port installed in your chest.'

Fucking hell. Anything else? Do you want to throw the kitchen sink at me, too?

Last time around, I was adamant I wasn't going to do anything that made me lose my hair. It was a non-negotiable to me. This time, I had to choose between my hair or going through hell again. Or dying. Not great options, whichever way you cut it.

'Do you have anything coming up this year we should be aware of?' the doctor asked later in our conversation.

'I'm getting married in ten months,' I said.

The look that flashed across his face was one of utter fear. I'll never forget his expression. It told me everything: *You may not have ten months.*

Voice of reason

Of course, he didn't say that out loud, but I'd become good at reading the cues. Sometimes silence speaks volumes.

I also spoke volumes in my first conversation with Dr T, and I was amazed at how deeply he listened to me. He took me seriously and didn't dismiss my thoughts or concerns. I hadn't had that from an oncologist before. I'd been saying how much I loved my surgeon and nurses, and soon I'd be able to say I loved my oncologist, too.

It was during this meeting that Dr T realised I had been allergic to a strand in the intravenous chemo which had made me so unwell. From my description of my reaction and the pure severity of the side effects, he gathered that my body clearly wasn't tolerating the oxaliplatin in the dosage. Dr T listed a 'moderate to severe allergy' on my medical records because it was the safest way to avoid it. I believe tests are required to get a clinical allergy diagnosis, but they understandably didn't want to test it on me to confirm because of how harsh my reaction was.

My treatment plan felt like a discussion, rather than a directive. Because of the trauma of my last experience with chemotherapy, I had a tower of mental blocks in front of me. By listening to me, Dr T knocked those blocks over and cleared the way.

He presented the medical non-negotiables, and I handed over mine. Number one: I couldn't do chemo at the same hospital anymore. It was too far away from my home, and the thought of 40 minutes of carsickness each way filled me with dread. Number two: I had to do chemo first thing in the morning. If I had an afternoon appointment, I would spend the morning stressing and getting worked up. I knew I needed to rip the bandaid off each day. Number three: my quality of life had to be considered. Always.

And so it became. The plan was for me to do chemo, of a morning, at a closer hospital, which was where Dr T worked and was only a ten-minute drive from my house. We agreed to see how the first dose of chemo went and alter accordingly as we went.

I don't know if telling people I had relapsed was harder than revealing my initial diagnosis. There was a lot of disbelief. 'I went into complete shock,' my friend Christina told me recently. 'I couldn't believe this could happen to such a young person. You just don't hear about it. Because it's not meant to happen. Your life was just beginning; you had a beautiful daughter and a whole future ahead. I didn't think it could be real.'

On 5 February 2023 I posted an update on Instagram, saying I was anxious as hell for the week ahead, but ready to get it over with. 'One foot in front of the other, one day at a time,' I wrote. 'Cannot freaking wait to live a carefree, healthy goddamn life!'

I wanted to get stuck in. Two weeks after my initial conversation with Dr G, I went into surgery to have my chemo port put in. Technically, you can start chemotherapy the day you have your port inserted, because it's just a funnel to your main line (vein). I thought back to the lady in activewear whom I met on my first day of intravenous chemotherapy—the first person I saw with a port installed. I remembered she looked so well.

I would have been kidding myself if I thought I could start chemo the day I had my port installed. It hurt. Like, it really fucking hurt. The incision in my chest was bad enough, but having a foreign implement in my body, under my skin, was uncomfortable and painful. I didn't have the energy to take my bandage off after the surgery, let alone be hooked up to a chemo machine.

Having the port was a bigger adjustment than I thought it would be. Unlike my stoma, I couldn't hide it as easily under clothes. I also couldn't have it reversed. It was going to be a permanent scar. My decolletage and my hair had been my favourite physical attributes. I loved wearing strapless outfits. I thought I wouldn't be able to do that anymore. I didn't want to show my port because it was an obvious sign I was sick and not 'normal'. But covering up and hiding parts of my body wasn't 'normal' for me, either. I felt self-conscious in my skin, to the point where I couldn't bring myself to take the padding off to look at the port.

At the time, the port felt like such a big deal. People tried to reassure me that it was just a scar, but it was more than just a scar to me. It was a battle wound from a fight I wanted no part in.

I started chemo a whole week after my port surgery. Compared to the previous treatment—which I was certain was going to kill me—this one was bearable. Little changes made the biggest difference. I was sensitive to all the beeps in the hospital, and my monitor beeped, so the oncologist and nurses let me turn it off to have a break from the triggering sounds. Instead of doing the infusion over two hours, we did it over eight, so it wasn't as harsh on my body.

I was on a two-week cycle, having an infusion every fortnight. I was slightly worried about that because my last rodeo was a three-week cycle, and I was a wreck for two weeks after each infusion before feeling okay for a week before the next one. I was scared I wasn't going to have any reprieve and that I would feel ill nonstop.

As you would expect, I felt pretty flat and deflated for the first couple of days after the infusion. But then I came good. I would go in on a Tuesday to start the infusion process, using my port and a portable pump that released the chemo over a couple of days. During those days, I didn't have to be in hospital and I could go about my business as 'usual.' The fatigue usually hit on Thursday, but come the weekend, I was—generally—doing okay. If Jeremy had a game or I had plans with friends, I could push through and forget about how I was feeling. It's a good thing I'm easily distracted, eh?

Voice of reason

I gave myself an almighty distraction when we decided to move our wedding forward. I hadn't been able to shake off the image of my oncologist's face when I told him I was getting married in October. We cancelled our original date not long after that conversation. I couldn't ask my loved ones to save a date I didn't know I would be around for.

Cancelling the wedding plans didn't make me want to get married any less. It was Mum who first suggested doing a pseudo-elopement: a small ceremony with our inner circle. Three weeks after putting the idea out there, Mum watched me walk down the aisle. I still can't believe we pulled it off.

As I've said, it wasn't the day I had dreamed of, nor the one we had originally planned, but it was everything it could have been. It's the moments that didn't go to plan that I remember the most. It was a windy day, and the arch we'd set up overlooking the beach was threatening to fall over. So Zac, who was Jeremy's groomsman, and his teammate Sam stood on either side of it to weigh it down during the ceremony. They're both big boys and were wearing white shirts, so they looked like my bouncers, standing guard. It was fitting considering there were legitimately paparazzi photographers hiding in the sand dunes taking photos of the wedding. We guessed that someone had tipped them off, or that we'd been followed from the hotel in the city where we'd all been getting ready. Sneaky.

The comical moments continued. Halfway through the ceremony, Sophia decided she wanted to feel the water and ran down the beach. My dad chased after her—even though he'd slipped over and broken his back a week prior—and struggled to keep up with her in the sand. It was quite the sight, an older fella in a suit chasing a toddler in a party dress. Poor Dad.

At the 'reception', which was more of a nice dinner, Jezz's dad, Gordon, decided to make a speech—even though we'd requested no speeches. He'd had a couple of beers by that point and was overcome with emotion when he started to speak. 'He's gone, our little boy,' he said through tears.

'You can have him back,' I joked. Everyone had a laugh.

We hadn't planned to 'announce' our surprise wedding so soon, but because of the paparazzi shots, we shared a photo on Instagram within an hour of saying 'I do'. We hadn't even had a chance to tell our wider group of friends and extended family before we made the public post. 'The Finlaysons', I wrote. The following morning I posted again, 'Feeling all of the love as we wake up as husband and wife this morning. Yesterday we got to say "I do" in such an intimate, romantic setting with the most intense love we've ever felt. We are extremely grateful for everyone that stepped up and made this happen, especially our parents, bridal party, brothers and sisters, for everything they've ever done, but most importantly for being there on a day we all thought would be so different and making it feel like we were exactly where we should have been.'

Voice of reason

Our hands might have been forced to make the announcement, but it wasn't all bad. We were showered in love, and even got an unexpected wedding gift from a local radio station. They called us the morning after the wedding and gifted us tickets to the Ed Sheeran concert the next night. It was such a whirlwind time. My first outing as Mrs Finlayson was to the Advertiser Foundation's Women of the Year Awards, where I was announced as 'Inspiration of the Year', and my second was to meet Ed Sheeran. We had a chat with him before his show, and he was so cool. His wife, Cherry Seaborn, had been diagnosed with cancer while she was pregnant with their second child. She had a tumour in her arm, which was removed a month after she gave birth. Ed understood more than most what we were going through.

I told Ed (I can call him that because we're mates) I used to live on Galway Avenue, and when he played the song 'Galway Girl' that night, he dedicated it to me. Then, when he changed his t-shirt before his last three songs, he gave me the shirt he had been wearing: a black tee with 'Adelaide' embroidered on it in rainbow colours. I posed for a photo holding the shirt, with the biggest smile on my face.

You would never have known I'd had chemo that morning. In fact, the Ed Sheeran gig was the first thing I'd done while attached to my chemo—the portable pump was hooked up to my port under my denim dress. Because the infusion had only started that morning, I didn't feel the effects until the next day. It was a bit of a nightmare; I was coming down from the adrenaline of the days gone by just as the chemo lethargy kicked in. Ouch. At least I had Ed Sheeran's tee to keep me company.

I ended up having six rounds of chemo, and there was only one that sat me on my arse. Of course, it happened to be the treatment before Easter. I was in Victor Harbor, an hour south of Adelaide, with Brya and her family, and my mum and Sophia. Jeremy had an away game in Sydney. Our dog had just had puppies, which was so exciting—especially for Sophia. We were using the opportunity to teach her about birth and give her the chance to help look after them. I couldn't give Soph a sibling, so this was the next best thing. We brought a stack of puppy pads with us on the quick trip down the coast. It was meant to be a weekend of puppies, babies and Easter eggs. It was all happening!

We left Adelaide for Victor Harbor on the Thursday night. I'd had chemo earlier that week. I was okay, until I wasn't. I started to feel off on Friday but pushed through. By Saturday, I was rat shit. Like, completely rat shit. We went for a walk down to a cafe to get coffee, but I couldn't eat breakfast. It was the sickest I'd been on the new treatment plan. I wasn't sure why; perhaps I hadn't taken enough anti-nausea medication.

I was so unwell, I put myself to bed and missed watching Jeremy's game on TV that night. His team was playing the

Voice of reason

Sydney Swans and it was a tight match. Jezz scored three goals and won the game for his team. In a post-game interview, the reporter asked Jeremy how he was feeling and mentioned my name. Jezz choked up. 'Yeah, I hope she's watching. I love her so much. This is the reward for sticking it tough and doing it for Kell and Soph back home. I'm just happy to be out here playing footy and doing what I love,' he said.

Of course it was the one game I missed. I woke up at 7 the next morning—having slept for fifteen hours—and I was delirious. I had no recollection of the night before. People would've been coming in and out of my room checking on me, and the puppies, and I didn't even stir. I was so glad that we happened to be with Mum and Brya so they could look after Sophia, because I was out of it.

When I checked my phone, I had dozens of messages and missed calls. *What the fuck has happened?* I thought.

'Omg, he's so beautiful,' someone wrote.

'What a good game! He's such a superstar!' said another.

A local radio producer reached out. 'How did you feel listening to the interview? Can we get you on the radio this morning to talk about it?'

There was too much noise. I had to put my phone in do not disturb mode. It would've been a lot to deal with on a normal day when I wasn't in the wars, but I was struggling to open my eyes. The only pain I can compare it to is a migraine. Everything felt heavy and blurry. I went back to sleep.

I woke up again at 11 a.m. to Sophia bringing me an Easter egg. It was Easter Sunday and I hadn't even realised. Soph had done her first Easter egg hunt without me. It was another milestone I missed out on.

It was then that I googled the game, saw the result and watched Jeremy's post-match interview. I bawled my eyes out listening to him speak so candidly about me on national TV. I was gutted to have missed the match and this moment. It was a major win for the team and a real milestone in their season. I should've been cheering my husband on, but I was out cold. I don't know what made me feel worse: the guilt or the crippling pain I was in.

It was the first time on my new regime that I questioned whether I could do it. *I don't know if I have it in me*, I thought.

And then the next morning, I woke up feeling . . . okay. Thank god! I *could* do it. I had to.

11
Not applicable

It felt like I was trapped in someone else's body. I was physically paralysed. My brain wasn't sending signals to my limbs. I wasn't in control. Something else had taken over.

I've never had anxiety before, so I didn't know what it was at first. The paralysis would take over en route to the hospital. Before that, even. It didn't matter if I was just going in for a routine appointment or a blood test. It wasn't rational; it was a trauma response.

My body would shut down. I would start hyperventilating and vomiting in the hospital carpark. I couldn't calm myself down. Even if I didn't think I was scared about whatever appointment I was going to, my body was terrified. My anxiety was a physical manifestation of the trauma I had been through.

I used to naively throw the term 'PTSD' around. 'Uh oh, I've got PTSD!' I would joke if I went to a restaurant where

I'd been with an ex-boyfriend. But PTSD is no joke. It's real and it's harsh.

It's true what they say: the body keeps the score. In the book by that name, written by Dutch psychiatrist Bessel van der Kolk, there's a quote the makes sense to me: 'When something reminds traumatised people of the past, their right brain reacts as if the traumatic event were happening in the present.'

You might think that, after nearly two years in and out of hospital, I would have become desensitised to it; that it would be my norm, that I could go to an appointment with my eyes closed. But the opposite was true. I grew more fearful of the hospital the more time I spent there. Merely walking through the oncology ward was incredibly triggering for me. Memories of my darkest days were down every corridor.

'You go to the hospital every two weeks. Aren't you used to it?' someone asked me.

No. I wasn't used to it. And I never would get used to it.

After the tough time I had over Easter, I told my oncologist about the reaction, and he lowered my dose to make it more manageable. Unlike the regime the year before, I was able to finish these six rounds. I went in for my twelve-week scan—to see where things were at before I started another six rounds—and there was no sign of the cancer in my stomach. The mass in my lung was still there, though. Instead of having to do another twelve weeks on the chemo, I was told I could have radiotherapy on my lung. It would be an intense dose, but I wouldn't have to do chemo during it.

The regime was direct radiotherapy, every two days for five rounds. Considering I had done 25 rounds of radiotherapy the year before—and handled it well—I thought it was going to be a piece of piss.

I was sitting in the radiotherapy waiting room when I heard an elderly woman's whisper. 'She looks far too young to be here,' the lady said, louder than she intended. She was right. Of course, yes, I was and am too young to be sitting in that room. I am evidently always the youngest in the oncology ward, usually by 30-plus years. It's uncomfortable having a room full of sad eyes trained on you. I know the other patients don't mean to pity me, but I can see it in their eyes.

The comment from the elderly woman in the waiting room was another reminder that people still believe that this is an old person's disease. I knew I had so much work to do to get the message out there loud and clear that cancer, no matter where the primary tumour is, doesn't care how old you are. That bowel cancer, the only cancer I have any experience with, is the leading killer cancer in 25 to 45 year olds. The woman's simple, innocent comment made me more determined to help people understand.

I became an ambassador for the Jodi Lee Foundation, which raises awareness of bowel cancer. Nick Lee created the foundation in 2010 after his wife, Jodi, died of bowel cancer. She was 40. She had two kids.

Like me, Jodi had been young, fit and healthy when she was diagnosed. There was no history of bowel cancer in her family, and her only symptoms were constipation, abdominal pain and some bloating, which could be chalked up to so many things. By the time the cancer was discovered, it had spread to Jodi's lymph and liver. It was too late to be cured.

There's a particular cruelty in knowing that if Jodi's cancer had been found earlier, it could have been treated. She could have survived.

Knowing how vital early detection is for bowel cancer outcomes, Nick created awareness campaigns, a national workplace program and fundraisers such as the Little Black Dress Ball. When I came on board as an ambassador I launched the Trust Your Gut campaign, encouraging everyone to listen to their body and seek help when things felt off. Part of the initiative was an online symptom checker to help people identify the signs of bowel cancer, which can be difficult to spot. I figured that if I could educate and motivate even one person to get checked for bowel cancer, something good could come out of the shitshow I was going through (no pun intended).

Being the poster girl for bowel cancer isn't the most glamorous title, but I felt proud to be raising awareness and sharing my story. I only wished I had a happy ending to share, too, but I only had a blank space. (Taylor Swift eat your heart out.)

Back to my own treatment: I don't know if I'm some kind of radiation superhero, but once again, I took it well. I didn't have any major side effects during the treatment. I had to wait six weeks after the last round before I could go in for another scan. When the time came, the results showed there was still cancer in my lung, but there had been a significant reduction and there was no activity. Whatever cancer was there was either dormant or dead.

'Fuck yeah! I won't have to do more chemo!' I meant to say this in my head; turns out I uttered it aloud. But then Dr T broke the bad news.

'Ah, yes you will. The cancer may be dormant, but it's still there. We want to make sure it doesn't come back. Let's do three more rounds.'

I gave Dr T his three rounds, but I negotiated with him every time.

'Alright, this time I'm only doing the infusion in the chair. I'm not having the pump,' I said during round two.

Eventually, Dr T realised I had switched off and that continuing with the chemo would do more harm than good to me. 'I know you're going to decline if you keep doing something that you're not mentally prepared for,' he told me. He was right. He knew me so well!

There Must Be More

It was July 2023 when I finished chemo. Things were stable. There was no activity on the PET scan, but the CT showed there was still a met (not a mass), a metastatic lesion, spread from the original tumour, in my lung. I went in and got my bloods done every two to three weeks to keep an eye on things. It was a matter of watch and wait.

I've never been much good at waiting.

~

'What is your prognosis?' the form asked me. Good question. I was filling out some medical paperwork and I didn't know the answer. I knew what my diagnosis was—Stage 4 colorectal cancer—but I didn't know what my prognosis was.

I called Dr G.

'Bro, what's my prognosis?' I asked.

'First of all, it's doctor, not bro,' he bantered with me.

'Yes, Doc. I'm filling out this form and can't find my prognosis in any of my paperwork. Where would it be?'

'I never gave you a prognosis,' he admitted.

'Why?'

'Well, you've already outlived it by more than a year.'

It was August 2023. I was first diagnosed in November 2021. I did the maths. My surgeon had initially predicted I only had six to nine months to live. He deliberately didn't tell me that.

Not applicable

'You know I've always been quietly confident. I never believed that prognosis to be the final story, and I knew you couldn't handle hearing it,' Dr G explained. 'I gave you every hard fact, symptom and side effect that you needed to know, but I never wanted to give you a timeline because I knew you would set yourself to that.'

Dr G didn't give me a death date for fear I would take his words as gospel. He knew if he told me I was going to die in six months, I would surrender to that knowledge and take it as the truth. So he didn't tell me. The man is very clever.

I realised I was alive because of his omission.

The news took a minute to sink in, when it did, I got back to the task at hand.

'So, what do I write on this form, where it asks for the prognosis?' I asked again.

'Just put n/a.'

Death is not applicable.

~

The headline screamed at me, and I wanted to scream back at it. The front page of Adelaide's *The Advertiser* declared in big, bold type: 'Kellie Finlayson: Cancer Free.'

It was news to me. And my mum, who was in a state. 'Why are people ringing me to say congratulations?' she asked, stunned and upset.

The night before, the TV program *The Project* had aired a segment with me and Jeremy. 'I'm one of the "lucky" unlucky ones,' I said in the interview with Georgie Tunny. 'My chemo is working so unbelievably well that my last scan was actually clear.'

The newspaper journalist had heard that quote—'my last scan was clear'—and taken it to mean I was cancer-free. They included the news on the front page, which I saw online the night before the printed paper came out. I rang them straight away. 'The headline is wrong,' I said. 'You can't print it.'

'It's already gone to print,' the person on the other end of the line told me. I felt unheard, misrepresented.

The misinformation was printed and distributed around Adelaide. Other outlets picked it up. My family members, friends and strangers read it. I received messages from dozens of people congratulating me on beating cancer. And I had to explain each time that it wasn't the case. I was not in remission. I still had cancer, but it was stable.

It hurt my mum the most. She was beside herself, having to explain to her friends and the lady at the bakery that her daughter still had cancer. Worst of all, she had to break the news to my aunties—her sisters-in-law—who had seen the headlines on Facebook. We had all dreamed about the moment I could say I was cancer-free, and for the newspaper to declare that I was—when I wasn't—was painful. We desperately wanted it to be true, but it wasn't.

I released a public statement correcting the newspaper's headline, but they didn't print a retraction or send me an apology. They revised their online headline, but it was too late: everyone had already seen it and shared it, and other media outlets had picked up the story, too It was clickbait bullshit, and all the clicks came at my expense.

I can see how someone might be confused about how my scans are clear, yet I still have cancer. Hell, it's confusing for me sometimes. It's a strange place to exist. I'm not a cancer survivor, because I still have cancer. I'm not a cancer patient, because I'm not in active treatment. So what am I?

I decided to coin a new description for myself: 'I'm a colorectal cancer thriver, not yet a survivor, but I'm working on it.'

Now that my cancer was stable, staying alive was no longer my full-time job. I genuinely could thrive instead of fighting to survive. You better believe that's exactly what I did.

Jeremy and I didn't get to go on a honeymoon. After our wedding in March 2023, I went straight back to chemo and Jezz went straight back to footy. We made up for lost time in October.

Going on an African safari was at the very top of my living list. It was the pinnacle. I had wanted to go on safari all my life, long before I was diagnosed with cancer. I set out to cross it off my list.

There Must Be More

We knew going on safari was a once-in-a-lifetime experience, so we decided to call it our honeymoon. I knew we shouldn't have to justify going on a holiday, but I felt better about the extravagance that way. We planned a two-week trip to Africa, using a generous wedding gift from my godfather, Uncle Mark, and his wife, Aunty Renee, along with all of our flight points.

It was just me and Jeremy. Sophia stayed in Australia, first in Queensland with Jeremy's family, and then with my mum at home in Adelaide, which was a holiday for Mum, too. We thought the flights and 2 a.m. safari start time might have been a bit much for a toddler, but as soon as we landed in Africa, we wished Sophia was with us. 'Omg, Soph would love this,' we both said on repeat.

We stayed in Zanzibar—where Freddie Mercury is from!—and swam in the pool, strolled on the beach and danced together at sunset. The safari itself was on mainland Tanzania. We woke up before dawn to travel deep into the wilderness, where we saw elephants, lions, giraffes, hippos and monkeys. It was straight out of *The Lion King*. All of my wildest dreams had come true. I was thankful for every second.

We left for Africa just after our original wedding had been scheduled. That wasn't lost on us. At the start of the year, we didn't know if I would still be alive in October, let alone in Africa! The timing made it all the more significant. I wasn't just alive, I was living.

Even during the trip of a lifetime on the other side of the world, cancer was ever present. The port in my chest and the wig in my suitcase were constant reminders. As I expected, I struggled with my hair loss. I first noticed it three rounds into the treatment. My hair started coming out in chunks when I brushed it. *Fuck, it's started*, I thought.

I didn't lose my hair all at once; it was a slow progression. I was self-conscious about it from the get-go. I noticed I wasn't going out as much, and when I did, I always wore a cap or a beanie. The only time I didn't have my head covered was at home, and even then, my hair was always up to disguise how little of it there was.

In July I was getting ready for a fancy gala, and I noticed my long-time hairdresser—Cole Tsakmakis at Coil Hair Studio (shout out)—was teasing the shit out of my hair. Usually she had to slick it back because it was so thick.

'How bad is it?' I asked.

'You've lost half of your hair,' she told me.

Luckily, I had plenty of hair to begin with.

The next time I was at the hairdresser—for another event—the trainee parted my hair to blow dry it. I looked in the mirror and gaped. 'Is that a bald spot?'

'Ah, yeah. You've got quite a few,' they said, gently.

I couldn't believe I hadn't noticed the bald patches. The spot in my part was only small, and when styled in a certain way it wasn't noticeable, but I could feel it. That day I had my hair cut the shortest it had ever been in my adult life. I actually loved it. I thought I looked like a 'cool mum'.

It wasn't until September—just before our honeymoon—that I went bald. Even then, I wasn't fully bald; I still had straggly bits. Because the process was so slow, I had months to come to terms with the loss, and months to research a good wig. I was very lucky I managed to get a real-hair wig at a discounted price. It still cost me $1000, but that's a bargain for a decent wig. The colour was identical to the hair I had lost. No one could tell the difference. I knew I was wearing a wig, but others didn't. The only difference was that the wig changed my head shape; other than that, it was indistinguishable from my former hair.

It took me a while to figure out how to wear the wig properly. There's a real art to putting a wig on and styling it. Once I got the hang of it, I felt better within myself. When I looked in the mirror wearing my wig, I saw me. My reflection was my own.

In Africa, I wouldn't leave the hotel room without my wig on, even if I was just going for a stroll. I know that's ridiculous—no one even knew me in Africa!—but I was so insecure, I couldn't bring myself to go out without my comfort blanket.

At the end of the trip, I posted a happy snap of me and Jezz on Instagram. I was wearing a cap. 'Coming home two shades darker, two kilograms heavier and two unbelievably grateful humans,' I wrote. 'We're so freaking happy to be on our way home to our little girl.'

Sophia wasn't the only thing that excited me about going home. I had a hair appointment booked in. I know, I know. Trivial, much? But after wearing a wig for a couple of months and watching my regrowth come through, I was ready to get extensions put in. My hair was patchy as all hell. The stuff that hadn't fallen out was longer and damaged, and the new growth was like alfalfa sprouts. The regrowth literally made me look like I had a mullet. Classy. My hairdresser worked her magic and somehow put extensions into my alfalfa sprout patch. They looked incredible, if I do say so myself. I was back, baby.

I was also excited to get home to launch a project that was close to my heart. I first heard about Sophie Edwards from nurse Paula, who had also introduced me to my friend Jordy. It was mid-2022, and Sophie was having a stoma put in after being diagnosed with Stage 3 rectal adenocarcinoma, a type of bowel cancer. I remember the first time Paula mentioned Sophie to me, because the name obviously reminded me of my Sophia. 'There's another young woman in the colorectal group,' Paula told me. 'She's pretty rattled.'

I knew the feeling. I found Sophie on Instagram, and we started messaging back and forth from our respective hospital rooms. We didn't actually meet in person at the time, but we became mates the old-fashioned way: on social media.

Sophie was going through the egg-retrieval process (which I couldn't have before I started treatment because my period hadn't returned after having Sophia). Sophie had a nine-year-old adopted son, but she hadn't experienced pregnancy or birth (and she knew when her last period was), so she was afforded the opportunity of egg collection.

When we did eventually meet in the real world, we realised we were basically the exact same person. Sophie and I had a ridiculous number of things in common. First up, we both had bowel cancer. Jinx. In addition to that, our parents were both adopted, and our mums were born on the same day, just different years. We were both December babies, and everyone had thought we were going to be born boys. More than anything, we both had the ability to talk underwater with a mouth full of marbles.

Sophie is seven years older than me, and right from the start I let her know it. If her wi-fi was playing up, I'd be quick to pass on my sympathies. 'It sucks to be old and out of touch with technology, hey,' I'd joke. If a song she liked came on the radio, I would feign ignorance. 'I've never heard this song. It must be from the eighties,' I would tease.

Sophie has become like a big sister to me. Sophia calls her Big Soph, playing on the fact that she's older than me, and Sophie jokes that she's the third partner in my marriage to Jeremy because she's always with us. We've formed such a close friendship. In fact, all of the friends I've made in the last three years have become really close. It's as though these friends have come into my life for a reason.

In so many ways, Sophie and I are kindred spirits. We bounce off each other and talk so much shit when we're together. Naturally, we decided to launch a podcast together, with help from our stoma sister Jordy. The name—*Sh!t Talkers*—works on two levels. We're literally talking about our shit and bowels, and also dribbling nonsense.

Sophie and I both thrive in the spotlight. We don't mind being the centre of attention or having an audience. I had built my own little community sharing my cancer experience, and Sophie had, too; we wanted to combine forces to unite our communities. Sophie had been on Season 4 of *The Bachelor* (the one with Richie Strahan), so she had her own profile. As a football wife (WAG), I had a bit of a profile, too, so we weren't strangers to the limelight.

In the months before I met Sophie, I had been a guest on so many podcasts talking about my diagnosis and treatment, but I hadn't come across a podcast dedicated to shitty situations. There's only so much you can share in a 45-minute interview on someone else's podcast. We wanted to tell the deeper stories. 'The good, the bad and the offensive' became our tagline.

It started with a live event: an 'in conversation' panel with Sophie and Jordy to raise money for the Jodi Lee Foundation. Originally, Jeremy had been on our list of speakers, along with

Sam Powell-Pepper, but the event was held when they were away at training camp. Regardless, the night went so well. We raised a few thousand dollars for the foundation, with enough left over that we could afford a set of podcasting gear. The team at the foundation encouraged us to keep speaking about our experiences. 'It's so educational and insightful hearing you all speak,' someone told me. 'It's a reminder that you're more than your disease.' That comment meant a lot to me. I know it's easy to judge others by looking at a picture-perfect, posed photo on Instagram, but photos never tell the full story. We wanted our podcast to show the reality of bowel cancer for the people who have it and the people who love them.

We launched our first-ever *Sh!t Talkers* episode on 27 December 2023. I introduced myself as, 'Kellie, also known as Jeremy Finlayson's terminally ill wife.'

'We're here to be a safe place, which we didn't have when we were newly diagnosed,' I explained. 'That is technically how we know each other—we've been through shit, grown through shit and done all the shit, but we also just want everyone to know that we are people outside our disease.'

Talking about shit can be uncomfortable, but Sophie, Jordy and I know all too well how important it is to push past the awkwardness and have these conversations. It wasn't all a selfless service, though: we also wanted to have a whole lot of fun. 'I reckon fun is the most prevalent thing that's going to come across. While, yes, we do have dark, deep conversations that are vulnerable, we are also funny as hell,' I said, oh-so humbly.

The podcast was a safe space for everyone, and Sophie was a safe space for me. I had stopped seeing a counsellor not long after I started. I tried therapy, but I didn't like it. In my sessions, I spoke about inconveniences and annoyances in my life, and avoided my feelings and worries, which I guess defeats the purpose of having a therapist. Sophie encouraged me to keep trying, to find the 'right' counsellor for me. But she basically became that herself. Sophie cops a lot of my trauma dumping. I'm open with her because she gets it.

Unless you've been touched by cancer, I'm not sure you have what's needed to guide someone else through it. Unless you've faced your own mortality—imagined your husband being a widower and your daughter growing up without a mum—it would be hard to put yourself in those shoes. Not that I would *want* anyone to put themselves in these shoes. They're uncomfortable as fuck.

Of course, people can be empathetic. They can offer strategies to help and give support, but they can't guide you down a path they've never walked themselves.

I'll admit that I probably do need to talk to a professional, but I know that will involve opening a lot of wounds, and I'm not ready to unpick those scars. I can talk about my experiences with Sophie on (and off) the podcast, and with strangers (when it has the potential to save someone's life), but I can't do it when the only motivation is myself. If the only reason to share is for me to understand my trauma more deeply, I'd rather not. Let's chat about something else.

When we started recording *Sh!t Talkers*, neither Sophie nor I were in active treatment. That would soon change.

12

Disguised blessings

The shortness of breath started when we got back from Africa. I tried to ignore it, to dismiss it, to will it away—but I knew something was wrong. I could feel it in my body. And yet, I didn't want to go to the doctor.

I was literally the face of a campaign promoting the 'Trust Your Gut' message, but I wasn't listening to my own. I was scared to trust my gut because I knew what it was telling me. It was whispering, warning me that I was back in the woods.

It was Sophie who pushed me to go and get a blood test. I had been having them fortnightly, but I hadn't had one since before going to Africa and I didn't have one booked in, so I rang up and made an appointment. I had my bloods drawn, and the doctor called me the very next day.

'Your levels are elevated,' they said, confirming what I already knew in my bones.

My tumour levels had been stable at 2 and they'd raised to 2.9. It was a small increase, but growth is growth. I was booked in for a scan, and had an anxiety-induced vomit in the carpark on the way to it. The results revealed that one of the mets in my lung (I had three all up) had grown by one millimetre. Another had grown slightly less than one millimetre.

I fucking knew it. God I hate being right all the time.

At the inevitable appointment with my oncologist, he told me we could still watch and wait, like we had been for the previous five months. The changes were small. We didn't need to panic. But when my next blood test came back at 3.6, I knew I couldn't wait around for the cancer to grow even more. 'I need to do something. I can't not,' I explained.

It was December 2023. My oncologist, Dr T, told me to spend Christmas and New Year's at home, and he scheduled me to start treatment in the first week of January. My treatment plan was another six rounds of chemotherapy. My hair had just grown back. I was not undoing the progress; I couldn't lose it again.

At the same time I was undergoing fertility tests, trying to sort things out in the hope of growing our family. I would've done anything to give Sophia a sibling. I had a hysteroscopy to check my uterus and cervix. It didn't look good. My uterine lining (where a baby would grow) was destroyed because of the radiation I'd had. We looked into buying donor eggs (at a cost of $30,000, with no guarantee they'd create embryos), but without a uterine lining, the eggs weren't much good to me.

Dr T gave me the option to protect either my potential fertility, or my hair. I chose my hair, after coming to terms with the fact that my fertility was highly unlikely to ever fix itself. Dr T tailored the dosage once more; it was less intense than what he'd given me the year before. No irinotecan (the strand that made me lose my hair), just the 5-FU, which was the bottle that I would wear home in my chemo pump for 48 hours after the initial infusion in the chair.

And so, I started 2024 in active treatment. For the fourth year in a row, I was a cancer patient.

It's a different experience the third time around. When I was first diagnosed, masses of people showed up for me. It was wild. My house became a florist, my fridge was full of lasagna and my phone was blowing up with calls and messages. People who I hadn't talked to in years, basically strangers, checked in. Everyone wanted to be kept in the loop.

Some of those people continued to check in, but many of them didn't. Perhaps because I was sharing so much of myself online, people might have assumed that if there was an update, they'd see it on Instagram. Others might have thought that, because I didn't die the first time, I'd be fine this time, too. I'd heard that this is a common occurrence; it's like people expect everything to return to normal after cancer. But, really, once you're diagnosed, you're never the same again.

Our sister-in-law, Jess, explained she got a jab of panic whenever I called her. 'I'm scared that this might be the call to say, "It's beat me,"' she told me. 'I get so scared thinking about a day when you might not be in the world with us, that I might lose one of my best friends and a sister, that I won't have anyone around to whinge about husbands and kids with.'

I, too, was scared of all of those things.

I don't know if I was just over it or if my mind and body were at their limit, but I couldn't cope with the chemo this time. I was deflated by the roller-coaster. I didn't want to be back in the chemo chair. I didn't want to be banned from kissing my husband. I didn't want to have my mum move back in with me to care for my daughter.

My dosage was lower than it had been, and I still couldn't tolerate it. I was a wreck, physically, but it could also have been a mental block. The beeping of the chemo pump made me feel like I was in hospital for the 48 hours I had to wear it at home. It was triggering—and knew that if my mental stability crumbled, my physical health would, too.

The silver lining of struggling so brutally with the chemo was that it made me look elsewhere for options. It was a blessing in disguise.

I gave my oncologist three rounds, and I wasn't even going to do the third round. I planned to call Dr T and tap out. I had a whole speech prepared in my mind. But when I was due to start, he was on leave so I couldn't call him. I couldn't get out of it. I had to push through.

I've never liked to say I'm 'fighting' cancer, because it's not a fair fight. If anything, it's a sucker punch from behind. I know 'fighting' is a commonly used term and part of our health vocabulary, but it doesn't sit right with me. To say someone 'lost their fight with cancer' implies that they're a loser, that they didn't fight hard enough, that they failed. It also implies that the only positive outcome is a win, a remission nod, a cure. Fuck that. Cancer isn't a win/lose situation. It's something people live with, manage and experience. And yes, it's also something some people die from.

Sure, every day of my life with cancer is a battle, but it's also a victory. I'm proof that you can live a full life with cancer.

The night before I jumped back into treatment, I posted a story on Instagram sharing that I was going to start chemotherapy again. Chemo was my only option. I had to take the post down the next morning because I was inundated with messages. So many of them were suggesting alternative routes. The people who wrote those messages mustn't have read the part that said chemo was my only option. As if I hadn't gone through every possible treatment idea, as if I hadn't researched other avenues, as if I hadn't read all the books and tried all the green juices, as if I hadn't done this twice before.

I know the messages came from a good place—people genuinely cared and wanted to help—but the tsunami in my inbox was overwhelming. I appreciated the messages of support, but I didn't appreciate the unsolicited medical advice or judgement.

∼

It was a harmless joke. I had a splitting migraine, no doubt because I was dehydrated and run-down. 'God, I hope I don't have a brain tumour,' I said flippantly to Jeremy who was beside me in bed. 'Let's hope I wake up.'

I promptly fell asleep.

It was the night before Rachel and Zac's wedding, and I needed my beauty sleep. So did Jezz—we were both in the bridal party—but he didn't get any. He was wide awake, worrying that I might actually have a brain tumour. I'd said it without a thought, but he couldn't stop thinking about it. The poor boy. He spent the next eight hours making sure I was still breathing and praying that I would, indeed, wake up in the morning.

I can't make those jokes anymore. I mean, I still do, but I shouldn't. Jeremy's reaction to my offhand comment reinforced that I will never be able to take my health for granted again. I will always be conscious of what is going on in my body. I will notice every little twinge and question every pain.

Once your health has taken such an enormous hit, any slight discomfort is taken seriously. If I have tightness in my chest, a headache that doesn't ease with Panadol or an ache in my back, my mind goes to a dark place. It's hard not to imagine the worst-case scenario, because so often I've been faced with exactly that.

For the rest of time, I will be hypervigilant.

I have a friend who says getting testicular cancer saved his life.

'Bro, make that make sense?' I said to him.

He told me that he'd been diagnosed, gone through treatment and been in the clear for five years when he started to feel that something wasn't right. He went to the doctor and that's when they discovered he had bowel cancer. If he didn't take that feeling seriously, he wouldn't have had a check-up, and they wouldn't have found the bowel cancer. It was so fast-growing, it would have killed him. Getting testicular cancer saved his life.

Anyway, I was relieved when I woke up without a migraine on the day of Rachel and Zac's wedding. And Jeremy was relieved I woke up at all! It was such a special day; she was the most beautiful bride and he was chuffed. It meant the world to me and Jezz to stand beside them. We had been through it all together; Zac was the first person I told about my pregnancy, Rachel was my maid of honour, they were Sophia's godparents.

There Must Be More

I love a wedding, and I loved this one a lot. It was a reminder of all the things I had to live for—love, family and good friends. Not that I needed a reminder. I knew exactly how much I had to live for every time I saw my daughter's face.

∼

In the time after my first relapse, I had started to research my diagnosis, different treatments and alternative routes in detail. I came across Hope4Cancer, a holistic care centre in Mexico for people with cancer and chronic illness. I followed a couple of people who had been to the clinic, and I reached out to one of them. Her name was Kate and she lived on the Gold Coast. She had been to Hope4Cancer twice for two separate cancers. She came back cancer-free both times. It sounded almost too good to be true. I had a million questions for her.

As it happened, when I spoke to Kate, she was back at the clinic sitting beside one of the nurses there.

'What would they suggest as an alternative treatment for a metastasised tumour in the lung?' I asked.

The nurse suggested sessions in a hyperbaric chamber, an infrared sauna and an LED red light therapy bed, as well as vitamin C drips. Of course, this suggestion was for my specific situation. There's a lot of controversy around vitamin C drips for cancer patients, so I had to do my research to make sure it wouldn't react with my tumour. I ran things by Dr T, and he was happy for me to explore my options as long as they weren't contradicting the treatment plan I was already on.

I was undergoing traditional Western treatment in hospital, and I wanted to do everything I possibly could to get things under control. I found a clinic on the Gold Coast that offered the alternative treatments I had been researching. Obviously, it wasn't viable for me to go there every week for appointments, so they put together an intensive program for me. The regime involved twice-daily sessions in the hyperbaric chamber, where I would spend an hour at a time.

I was so lucky to have dear friends on the Gold Coast (whom I met in the AFL hub during Covid restrictions) with a massive property, including a little house that they listed on Airbnb. Without hesitation, my friends offered me the house for the week, which saved me thousands of dollars and meant I could fly myself, Mum and Sophia up.

Remember how I said it felt like all of the friends I'd made in years gone by were meant to be? That they came into my life for a reason? Yeah, I'm sure this is one of those cases. There's so much I couldn't have done without my friends' support.

I know it's a privilege to be able to fly three people across the country for a week, but it felt necessary to me. At that point in time, we were back to not knowing how many days I had left, so I didn't want to spend a single day without my daughter if I didn't need to. I wanted her with me. And I needed Mum's help.

With Mum's support, my friends' kindness and Sophia's strength, I went hard for five days, having sessions twice a day. The treatment itself was physically easy. It involved equalising as the pressure within the chamber intensified, and then watching hours of Netflix each time. But the intense pressure was exhausting—it was like deep-sea diving—and after a few days in a row, I was spent.

If I hadn't found these resources in Australia, I would have been seriously considering a stint at Hope4Cancer in Mexico. We did the maths, and it was going to cost us $90,000. That was before looking at prices for flights and accommodation for Mum and Soph, because there was no way I was spending a month away from them.

When I got back to Adelaide from the Gold Coast, I had a blood test. The results were astonishing. In the span of two weeks—after my last chemo infusion and my week on the Gold Coast—I had halved my tumour levels. They went from 6.9 to 3. Anything under 2.5 is healthy, under 5 is normal and above 5 is serious. I'd gone from serious to normal, verging on healthy.

'Holy shit, it's working,' Dr T said. He had always been open to alternative options—I remember trying to convince him that worming tablets might be worth looking into because I'd read an article on them, and he didn't tell me to shut up—but this really showed what a difference they could make. (Also, it's worth noting, I do take a small dose of fenbendazole—which is used in worming tablets—in one of my prescriptions, so I wasn't entirely wrong about that.)

I knew it wasn't feasible to fly to the Gold Coast every fortnight or month, so I kept researching and found someone in Adelaide with a hyperbaric tank. I had already looked into using the one at the hospital, but they wouldn't take me because I'd had a collapsed lung in the past. The medical grade tank at the hospital would've been too extreme for me and would've made me a liability for them. The one I found was called an Airpod, and I learned people use them to regenerate their blood flow. Essentially, it oxygenates your blood so cancer can't live in it. In that scenario, the chemo treatment I was having was able to attack the cancer with the upper hand. The Airpod worked well in conjunction with the treatment I was already undertaking. It wasn't a miracle cure, but I found it helpful and saw the benefit of it.

I wish these alternative treatments were talked about more. I know it's important not to give false hope or make unsubstantiated guarantees—Belle Gibson, the cancer fraud who claimed green juices cured her, really fucked things up for the rest of us—but silencing all avenues that are outside the box isn't helpful. I don't think it needs to be one or the other. I think Western medicine and alternative treatments can exist in the same regime.

These experiences were my first real insights into the world beyond Western medicine. I always knew there must be more. And I was right. Standard.

There Must Be More

I hope you know my arrogance is mostly ironic. It's a coping mechanism for me. I take the piss, I crack a joke, I break the ice. There's so much heaviness in my world, I need moments of levity. Sometimes my jokes might not be appropriate, but there's nothing appropriate about cancer. It's fucked. My humour might be dark, but so is what I'm going through.

I know not everyone will 'get' my disposition, but please know, I'm doing my best.

~

I was desperate to see Taylor Swift on the Australian leg of her Eras tour. As was every other bloody person in the country. They were the hottest tickets in town, and I didn't have one. I could blame the uncertainty of cancer for not planning ahead, but it wasn't just the cancer. So many people missed out on tickets because they sold out so fast.

I was in the thick of active treatment when Tay Tay arrived Down Under, but I was determined to see her live. A dose of glittery, girl-power goodness was exactly what I needed. I posted on my Instagram Stories asking if anyone was selling Taylor Swift tickets. I wasn't asking for a freebie; I just wanted a lead on a ticket for sale. The story got heaps of shares and comments, and I was hopeful the universe would provide.

Disguised blessings

Then I got a DM. It was from someone I went to school with. As soon as I started reading the message, I knew he hadn't meant to send it to me. He had forwarded me my own Story with the message. It was about me, but it wasn't for me.

'I can't fucking stand that she's using her illness to get free tickets to Taylor Swift,' he wrote.

'Huh?' I replied. 'Clearly not meant to be sent to me.'

He unsent the message. It didn't matter. I'd already seen it.

'Thanks for bitching about me behind my back,' I wrote.

He blocked me.

He wasn't getting away with it that easily; I messaged his wife. 'Let him know I saw his messages, and I don't appreciate it,' I wrote. 'I hope he's never touched by a chronic illness.'

He replied.

'Okay, I'm sorry, that was fucked. What I was meaning was that I was annoyed that someone in your position with your platform that you normally use for amazing work regarding cancer, was using it and asking people to give you tickets. I'm sorry, it was a dick move and I do feel terrible,' he said.

I wrote back, via his wife, because I was still blocked.

'I'd like to highlight that not once was I asking for someone to give me tickets,' I wrote to her. 'I was in fact trying to buy tickets from someone who can no longer go or has tickets available. Not that I have to justify or explain myself, because what I put on a platform that I do indeed use for the most selfless reasons, advocating and saving other people's lives, while I can't even save my own, I'm allowed to be selfish every now and then. I'm offended. I'd love to understand what he meant by me being in the position I'm in, because the last time I checked that position isn't one I ever wanted to be in.'

His message gutted me, but I know he's not the only one who thinks that way. I would never have chosen to get cancer. And I certainly would never have chosen to get cancer in exchange for publicity, Instagram followers or PR freebies. As if. I only started sharing my experiences on social media because I thought it might help others. It might encourage someone with worries to get checked, or make someone with cancer feel less alone, or inspire someone in the trenches to advocate for themselves.

Putting yourself—your scars, stories and life—on the internet isn't for the faint-hearted. It's a vulnerable thing to do, opening up to strangers and baring your soul. Originally I was sharing for loved ones, making it easier for me to relay an update to hundreds of friends checking in, I didn't do it for myself, though the deep sense of connection I felt from others going through a similar feat was weirdly comforting. I did it for all the other young girls out there thinking they have a gluten intolerance when they actually have bowel cancer and need to get a colonoscopy. That's the thing, with everything I do, I expect feedback, and it's not always going to be positive, which is unfortunate, but I also have a deep sense of self-worth and know that not everyone is going to agree with the way I go about things. I know that choosing to keep my illness to myself would seem easier, it would reduce judgement, but it would also reduce the number of lives I'm able to save. I wish I could explain the obligation I feel to make a really shitty diagnosis have an incredibly powerful outcome. I found comfort in knowing that the more I share, the more of a positive impact I'm able to make, the more people I can reach, the more lives I can save.

Cancer is shit. It's the worst. I didn't want it and I certainly didn't choose it, but I do try to make the best of the card I've been dealt. I try to find the silver linings. Fuck, I try to *be* the silver lining.

So criticise me for wanting to see Taylor Swift!

In a move that I hope royally pissed off my old school mate, I managed to get a ticket to one of Taylor's Melbourne shows. I put on a floral mini dress, gold heels and a cowboy hat, and I sang my little heart out. I was up close near the front of the stage having the time of my life, and I swear Taylor looked straight at me and smiled. We had a moment.

It was a show I'll never forget; a much-needed reprieve from my reality. And a reminder that some dickheads from high school never grow up.

There Must Be More

I found Dr N on Google, while I was still hooked up to my chemo pump, going through my third round. Dr N is a holistic health naturopath, specialising in many of the alternative treatments I'd been reading about—particularly Oncotherm, which is all about applying a focused electromagnetic field to target only the cancerous cells (they have higher conductivity) and deep heat them to stimulate the body's immune response and trigger the cells' self-destruction. At our appointment, I had a big, cold plate attached to my chest. The plate was hooked up to a machine. When it was turned on, the plate heated my insides. I swear to god, it felt like my cancer was burning up. I could pinpoint pain where I knew my mets were located. I know it might have been in my head, but I could physically feel it working—it felt like the plate was heating the chemo and killing the cancer faster. You don't have to be undergoing chemo to use the Oncotherm, but they work well in conjunction.

Dr N put together a health program for me. It involved doing cycles of a keto—low-carb, high-fat—diet, to starve my cancer of the glucose it needs to survive, as well as taking certain supplements, and undergoing pulsed electromagnetic field (PEMF) therapy, which sends energy pulses through the body to improve bloods.

I also started doing ozone saunas, in a machine that looked like a little rocket ship with space for my head to pop out at the top. The aim of this machine is to warm up your core temperature—minus your head—to a high heat while pumping ozone gas into your skin, to boost your immune system. As if that wasn't enough, the heat is also designed to cause your body to sweat out toxins at the same time. They suggest sitting in the ozone sauna for 45 minutes, but I usually only made it to 30. It didn't hurt, it was just fucking hot.

I am conscious of talking about the particular therapies I've done or am doing, because I am not a doctor. These are all things I've found through my research or via my health practitioners. They're things that I've been willing to try and have found helpful. That might not be the case for everyone.

I would never claim to be a cancer expert, because my expertise is specific to my cancer, my body, my research. I wouldn't dream of suggesting treatments for other people. The only thing I would recommend is to do your own research, to take your time and to get a second opinion. When it comes to something as important as our health, we should all take the time we need to make decisions. I remember the pressure I felt immediately after my diagnosis to make decisions and start treatment. If I could go back and tell younger Kellie one thing, it would be this: 'Don't rush into anything. Regardless of how urgent it feels in the moment in the doctor's office, you have more than two minutes to decide what you want to do. Go home and think about it. Give yourself twenty-four or forty-eight hours. Don't sign the paperwork straight away. Take some time.'

There Must Be More

After my third round of chemo, I had 'the talk' with Dr T. I was done. He knew it and I did, too. My inflammation levels were at 2.2, which meant they were healthy, so he booked me in for a scan to take a closer look. The results showed my mets were stable and had shrunk. There was something else interesting on the scan: the mets looked hollow. Like little donuts, only less delicious. Dr T hadn't seen anything like it.

Once again, he told me to keep doing whatever I was doing. It was working.

13

One foot in front of the other

I hit the bitumen like it had wronged me. It was dusk, and I was running for the first time in three years. I didn't tell anyone what I was doing. I just put my trainers on, grabbed my earphones, walked out the front door and went for my first run since I'd found out I was sick. I slammed the door on my way out. The run was fuelled by frustration. I was pissed off about something—life!—and I needed to get it out of my system. I didn't want to sit on the couch and wallow; I wanted to run.

Up until that moment, I had been too afraid to run. I was worried about my lung capacity and how my body would hold up. But I was also scared of disappointing myself. I thought if I couldn't run a certain distance, I would be a failure.

It took getting mad to get back out there. *Just see how far you can go*, I told myself. *The worst thing that will happen is you'll get a tight chest and have to walk.*

I ran for 3 kilometres. It was hard. Like, *really hard*. But I did it.

Jeremy thought I'd just ducked out to the shop around the corner to grab something for dessert. When I came home without dessert, all hot and sweaty, he realised I'd been for a run. 'Holy shit, you must have been angry, babe,' he said, knowing me well.

I left the anger on the pavement. It was such a release. I didn't realise how much I had missed running.

～

It was in Norway that I started running regularly. I ran to clear my head, to get my heart rate up, to push myself. While I was living in Arendal, I started a Parkrun group there with a few of my colleagues—and as far as I'm aware, it's still going today. I remember starting a run wearing multiple layers in the cold and stripping them off as I went. There was something satisfying about outrunning the cold.

Exercise became my best friend while I was living overseas. Keeping fit really helped with my mental health. I didn't have many homesick moments, but I relied on running and working out to distract myself when I did. After six months of living—and training—in Norway, I entered my first half marathon, without knowing what I was signing up for. The furthest I'd run before that was 8 kilometres. A half marathon is just over 21 kilometres.

One foot in front of the other

My friend Josh Lynott—from Australia—was hosting a mindset retreat in Siargao, the Philippines, which involved running, clearing rubbish in local communities and raising money for charity. There were about ten of us there from all over the world, including another girl from Norway and one from Sweden, whose name was Sofie (pronounced Sophia). Only a couple of people in the group had run long distances before, so it was a learning curve for all of us. We started off doing 5 kilometre runs, up and down hills.

On the morning of the half marathon we woke up at 4.30 a.m. and had a coconut coffee (when I tell you I still dream about this tastiness, it's—not a word of a lie—delicious) and rice crackers with banana and peanut butter for breakfast. Josh warned us not to fill up too much. We were on a mission.

I partnered up with Sofie, who had only ever run 5 kilometres, and we ran together. My mission was to get her through it, a bit of a theme throughout my life is clearly to forget about my pain in order to help others through something, ironic. I wasn't thinking about myself, until we hit the 15-kilometre mark. That's when I started to slow down. Slowing my pace affected my rhythm and made every step feel harder. I knew I had to pick up my pace to make it, and that's what I did. The last 1.5 kilometres were up a steep incline, and the end of the run was on a plateau, surrounded by fields. It felt like I was running above the palm trees. It was incredible.

There Must Be More

I didn't feel any pain until I stopped. When I jumped on the back of a scooter to get back to our resort, I was sure my hip flexors would never forgive me. By the time I made it to my room, I couldn't move without wincing in pain. Everything hurt.

It didn't matter. I was on an almighty high. Just like that, I was a runner. I went on to do half marathons in Istanbul, Berlin and Melbourne. I was running half marathons on a Sunday in Norway. For fun! Who was I!? I would literally get home from a 20-kilometre run, take a dip in the freezing-cold lake, lie out in the 12 degree sunshine (warm for Arendal), then spend the day with my friend Lorelei exploring different parts of our 'home'. I was a proper athlete: training, recovering and beating PBs (that means personal best, FYI—something I learned along the track). It is so strange to look back on how fit I was during that time.

Just like travelling, I thought running would always be a part of my life.

It's not until something is taken away from you that you truly realise how much it means to you.

～

Running is brutal. I don't think anyone actually likes running when they're running. You feel great afterwards, but in the moment, it sucks.

One foot in front of the other

After dusting my trainers off when I stopped chemotherapy in March 2024, I did my first 5-kilometre run with the Lambros brothers—Lachlan and Stefan Lamble—who were running across Australia raising money for cancer research. I joined them on the Adelaide leg of their trek from Perth to Melbourne. At the 700-metre mark, the boys (who were fit as fuck) were still chatting to me while we were running.

'Guys, I can't run and talk, it's one or the other,' I said.

There were a few moments in which I questioned if I could finish the 5 kilometres. When I said as much to the boys— 'I don't know if I can do this'—they were totally blasé about it. 'Yeah, you can,' they said, without hesitation.

That used to be me. I used to be the one telling others that they could absolutely keep going. 'You'll be fine. It's not that hard. Just put one foot in front of the other,' I would say.

I wasn't used to being the one struggling and needing encouragement, but the boys cheered me on, and I did it.

A month later, in May, Lachlan and Stefan became the first brothers to run across the country. They raised over $238,000 for cancer research.

I don't know if I'll be able to run long distances again. I always used to say that it was harder to run 3 kilometres than it was to run 10, because after the first 3 you settle into a rhythm and your body takes over. But that's an easy statement to make when you're in your early twenties, without a kid or a terminal illness. If I were to go on a run with my younger self today and heard her tell me to just put one foot in front of the other, I'd probably tell her to go jump.

I've been taking things one step at a time since my world came to a standstill in 2021. Some days, one step is all I can manage.

I knew regaining my fitness wouldn't happen overnight. Even though I had stopped chemotherapy, I was still immunocompromised. I wasn't as strict as I had been about avoiding sickness when I'd first been diagnosed, because I couldn't be. Soph was in daycare, and germs are part and parcel of that. Some people might question why I'd risk having her in daycare when the chance of catching something is so high, but it's so important to me for Sophia to spend time with other kids. She has the cutest little friends at daycare and in her extracurricular classes, and I wouldn't dream of taking those friendships away from her. She is a social butterfly, and it would be enormously selfish of me to dull her shine or take away opportunities out of fear.

Sophia has spent too much of her young life in and out of hospital with me. Her earliest memories are tainted by the scent of medical-grade antiseptic. I don't know how aware she is of my health. We call my chemo port my 'owwies', to help her understand why I might be feeling unwell when I'm undergoing treatment. I'll never forget the moment Soph was sitting on my lap as I was having blood drawn, and she asked,

'Why they want Mummy's blood?' How do you answer that question in an age-appropriate way?

I told Soph they were making sure my blood was nice and healthy. I don't know if that was the right answer. It's such a fine line between being honest and scarring your child for life. I want to protect Soph at all costs, but there's only so much I can shield her from when this is our reality.

We are lucky that Soph is the world's most resilient toddler. She doesn't know any different. If someone's sick or injured, she refers to them 'being sick like Mummy' or 'going to doctor like Mummy'. She understands that I'm not well but she has no concept of just how unwell I am. I recently overheard Soph explaining to Frankie (Brya's daughter) that Mummy was having a sick day on the couch, so they should play upstairs while I rested. I've heard her tell people, 'Mummy has a really sick tummy' or 'Mummy hurts to breathe.'

On the days I don't make it out of bed, Soph brings her dolls to me, or recruits Grandma to play with her. She knows when I need to rest, but I don't think she realises it's any different to when Jeremy has a hangover.

I'll always keep her knowledge of my health relevant to her age. She doesn't need to be aware; she needs to be a child.

When I dropped Soph off at daycare one day, I told her I was off to see the doctor and I'd see her later that afternoon. When I picked her up, the first thing she did was check the port in my chest to see if anything had been attached to it.

She was relieved when it hadn't. I hate that my port is something she's aware of, but it's normal for her. Soph knows she can't share the same cup as me because of how toxic my chemo is. 'Naughty medicine,' she calls the tablets I have to take.

I think the biggest impact my health has had on Soph is her having several parental figures: me, Jezz and my mum, plus all the other people in our lives who've stepped up and taken care of her. Because she's spent so much time with adults—not just me and Jezz—her cognitive function is extremely advanced for her age. She'll hang out with basically anyone, which makes life a hell of a lot easier if we need someone to help out for a few hours here or there.

Cancer is a thief. It steals time, moments and memories. The biggest thing cancer has taken from me is my fertility. It was such a blow being told I didn't have time to go through the egg-retrieval process before starting treatment. If I'm honest, I'm still reeling from it.

Jeremy and I always wanted three kids: two girls and a boy. Jeremy was one of four, and I was one of two, so three was straight down the middle. When we pictured our life together, we saw ourselves with three little ones, a happy family, bursting with love.

Being infertile is something I haven't come to terms with, and I don't know if I ever will. I know infertility is an extremely sensitive subject; so many families struggle with not being able to fall pregnant easily (or at all), and I acknowledge how privileged I am to have had Sophia. I count my lucky stars for my daughter every day. She is my purpose in life, and I will live all of my days for her. As blessed as we are to have Sophia, though, it still stings not being able to have the family that we envisioned, and having to grieve the life we had planned.

Infertility in peak motherhood age is especially cruel. I have an intense sense of desperation, like my body wants to be pregnant, but it physically can't be. The feeling of failure is excruciating. I've struggled watching (seemingly) everyone around me get pregnant and grow their families without issues. I've choked back tears seeing mums with newborn babies walk down the street. I've pretended to be okay—and even happy—when I've felt depressed and despondent. Every pregnancy announcement on Instagram has been a dagger to my heart.

~

I've always wanted to adopt a child. Because both my parents were adopted, I grew up knowing that there's more than one way to have a family. You don't have to be blood related to be family.

When I was around twelve, Mum signed up for the TV show *Find My Family* and found her biological mum and stepdad, but she still doesn't know who her father is. It wasn't an easy thing to do.

My dad has never tried to find his birth family. He knows he has two brothers in Whyalla—the small town where he was born, north-east of Port Lincoln—but he's never tried to meet them. It's wild to me; Dad often goes to Whyalla because there's a motorsport track there, and he is heavily involved in racing. There have been so many times when Dad has been called another name while visiting Whyalla. I'm sure he was being mistaken for one of his brothers. I couldn't stand not knowing where I came from, but Dad is content with the parents who raised him and the sister he grew up with (who was also adopted). He doesn't have any urge to dig deeper. Of course, that's entirely his choice.

Adoption rates peaked in the early 1970s, just after my parents were born. There were different societal expectations back then: unwed mothers were pressured into adopting out their babies, and closed adoptions were preferred because it was assumed that a 'clean break' from the biological mother was best. According to the Australian Institute of Health and Welfare, in 1971–72, almost 10,000 children were adopted in Australia. In 2022–23, there were 201 adoptions in Australia.

It's a hard, lengthy and expensive process to adopt in this country. Still, Jeremy and I were willing to do whatever we needed to. But, after starting to investigate the process, we found out that we were not allowed. I have a big red mark against my name. Because I am terminal, I'm not eligible to adopt. Jeremy could adopt on his own as a single parent—which would be hard—but we couldn't do it as a couple because of my health.

Once again, cancer had taken something from me: the ability to adopt a child.

~

It was my neighbour's seven-year-old daughter, Alessia, who first suggested the idea. My neighbour, Christina, had just had her third baby and I was as clucky as anything. I must have said something about wanting another baby.

'Why don't you have one, then?' Alessia asked me.

'Oh, sweetie. My oven is broken so I can't,' I told her, in simple terms.

'That's okay, just use Mum's oven, it works fine,' she said, as though it was such an obvious solution. Duh, Kellie.

She was on to something, though. I hadn't considered surrogacy until the seven-year-old next door suggested borrowing someone's oven.

And so, I delved into the unknown depths of surrogacy in Australia. I did all the research, read all the articles, followed all the TikTok accounts and joined all the Facebook groups. That's when I saw a post from R, who was interested in becoming a surrogate. Her name and face looked familiar. I clicked on her profile, and we had dozens of friends in common. She was from the Eyre Peninsula, too; I had played netball with her older sister. Small world, eh? So small, I decided to add R as a friend, and she sent me a message.

I learned that R had a nine-year-old daughter, and she didn't want any more kids of her own, but she did want to experience pregnancy again. R had fallen pregnant when she was seventeen. She gave birth three days before her Year 12 formal. She didn't get to enjoy her pregnancy or birth because she was so young, stressed and scared. R knew pregnancy could be beautiful, and she wanted to experience it like that. She wanted to be in control, rather than the situation being in control. She wanted to write her own narrative and bring life into the world on her own terms. But she didn't want a baby herself. R was more than content with her daughter, who was thriving as an only child.

There was something comforting and reassuring about R's desire to be a surrogate. She was in it for the right reasons. Jeremy and I had been worried that someone might offer to be our surrogate for the wrong reasons—to be blunt, for Jeremy's sperm. As an elite athlete with a high profile, it wouldn't have been out of the realm of possibilities for someone to do such a thing. We had to consider whether a surrogate would try to run off with the baby.

One foot in front of the other

When we met R, though, we knew we didn't have any cause for concern. For one, she's an incredible human who strongly believes in good karma. Also, she has no idea about AFL. I'm not joking. Before we met, R didn't have a clue that AFL players are paid. She thought the game was just something boys did on the weekend. She didn't realise being in the AFL was a full-time job. When Jeremy was sidelined with an injury, she was worried about him not getting paid for an uncertain amount of time.

'Oh, you poor thing. It must be hard with him being off work for so long. Are you going to be okay financially?' she asked.

'Um, Jeremy still gets paid for training and recovery. He's a full-time employee.'

I saw the realisation spread over her face.

R is quite literally one in a million. Not only did she offer to be our surrogate, she also donated her eggs. Since I didn't have time to undergo the egg-retrieval process before I started treatment, I don't have eggs of my own. Of course, using R's eggs and Jeremy's sperm meant they would be the baby's biological parents. Naturally, that knowledge was a bit tough for me to take on.

Then I met R's daughter, who has blonde hair, blue eyes and olive skin. I swear she looks exactly like an older Sophia. After that, I was more confident that the baby would still look like Sophia, which put me at ease. I would be the baby's mum,

Jeremy would be the dad, Sophia would be the big sister and R would be our very generous surrogate.

Sophia began calling R 'Aunty Shell', and saying, 'Aunty Shell is making me a baby.' It was the sweetest.

The surrogacy process started with lots of red tape and paperwork. Both us and R had to retain legal counsel. R's lawyer had been a surrogate herself, so she understood the experience better than most. I googled 'surrogacy lawyers in Adelaide' and came up blank. Instead, I found a family law practice and noticed one of my old school mates was a lawyer there. I messaged her on Instagram to ask if she knew anything about surrogacy contracts and, as luck would have it, she'd just finished her first surrogacy case. I told her in the strictest confidence that we were hoping to have a baby via surrogacy, and we retained her services to write up the agreement. Because we knew each other, I felt more comfortable messaging her with questions along the way and she helped us through every step.

Next up we had to go through a series of counselling sessions. They were as confronting as they were insightful. One of the first questions R was asked was, 'If Kellie and Jeremy die in a car accident the day after you fall pregnant, are you going to keep the baby?' The question threw her, and she mumbled something about that not happening. She rang me straight after the session. 'Please tell me you have a will drawn up?' she said.

One foot in front of the other

'Of course! We have things in place if anything were to happen to me or Jeremy,' I reassured her.

When Jeremy was asked the elephant-in-the-room question—'Are you scared Kellie won't be around to see the baby grow up?'—he answered honestly. Of course he was.

We both hoped that his honesty hadn't ruined our chances of becoming parents via surrogate.

When we started looking into having another baby, I didn't question whether growing our family was a selfish dream. It is something I've thought about since then, though. People—strangers—have questioned how I can bring a new life into the world not knowing how much life I have left. It's a fair question. And, for a while, the question stopped me from moving forward.

But here's the thing: we're all going to die. No one knows how long they have left. Any one of us can be hit by a bus tomorrow. If we all let the fear of death stop us from having kids, the human race would die out.

I've spent a lot of time reflecting on whether it is selfish for me to want to have another child. Ultimately, it was a comment from an only child that made the decision for me. 'I'm never going to be an aunty,' the woman told me, with sadness in her voice.

I adore Jeremy's nieces and nephews, and my friends' kids who I'm a pseudo-aunt to. It broke my heart to think of Sophia being deprived of that—of not having a sibling now, or nieces and nephews later.

There Must Be More

There are so many unknowns in life, and there will never be a right or wrong answer when it comes to starting or growing a family. But personally, I believe that giving Sophia a sibling is what's best for our family—regardless of whether I'm in their life for a long or short time. Everyone's parents die. It's inevitable. But when you have a sibling, you can go through the loss together. Giving Soph a brother or sister feels like the least I can do for her.

14

A non-ideal world

The sound was like a balloon squeaking as it deflates, except it wasn't coming from a balloon—it was coming from inside my body. It was mid 2024, and I had pneumonia. I was struggling to breathe. That's not unusual when you have pneumonia, but the sound was unusual. It happened on the depth of my breath. When I inhaled and exhaled deeply, I became a squeaky toy.

I messaged the Port Adelaide club doctor (a perk of being 'Jeremy Finlayson's terminally ill wife'), and he got me in for an X-ray. Nothing showed up on the scan. Like, not even the pneumonia. The doctor said my chest looked good (not in *that* way). There was no congestion or visible reason for the squeaking sound when I breathed. I started a course of anti-inflammatory medication and steroids and hoped that would be the end of it.

In the meantime, I had a long-awaited appointment with my surgeon, Dr G. Because I had been stable for so long, I was desperate to have surgery to remove the mets in my lungs. I wanted them out of my body: gone, goodbye. I wasn't a doctor (obviously), but I knew it could be done because others had had the surgery. I wanted to know if and when I could have it, too.

Dr G knew I wasn't going to let the idea go, so he took my case to a multidisciplinary meeting with other specialists. His concern wasn't the surgery itself, but what it could trigger. After a surgery, when your body is healing, things grow back—the tissue, skin, certain organs and microscopic cancer cells. Dr G didn't want to wake up the cancer cells or give them an opportunity to grow. Still, he was willing to refer me to a lung surgeon (who had a reputation for being aggressive in his methods), on the condition that I had a PET scan first.

I hadn't had a PET scan in months because my CT scans were so stable. The PET scan would show if the cancer cells were active. If they were not active, he wouldn't recommend the surgery because it would be asking for trouble. If that were the case, I was prepared to follow Dr G's judgement—and sit still. 'If there is activity, though, I get my way?' I bargained.

It was a classic case of 'be careful what you wish for'. The PET scan revealed I had several growths. The growth in my mets was less than a millimetre, but it was there, and that wasn't good news.

A non-ideal world

After the PET scan, I found out my lung had collapsed in three places, which explained the squeaking noise when I breathed. One collapse was thanks to the scar tissue left over from radiation, and another was from the growth of one of my mets. I wasn't worried about the collapsed lung—I'd had one before and it wasn't a big deal, it just made it harder to breathe—but I was worried about what effect it would have on my chances of surgery.

I made appointments with my radiotherapist, my holistic oncologist and the lung surgeon, in the hope that they would suggest an option that didn't involve chemotherapy. My radiotherapist didn't recommend more radiation because it would only create more scar tissue which would lead to more lung collapses. My holistic oncologist put me on a new trial, which didn't have concrete results yet, so it wasn't a guarantee. And the lung surgeon gave me some odds. 'I'm sure I can get ninety-nine per cent of the mets in the surgery,' he explained. 'But I'm one hundred per cent sure that the one per cent left over will grow when you're healing.'

Fuck.

The lung surgeon ruled surgery out. He told me what I already knew but was desperately avoiding: I needed more chemo. But he assured me that if I did six months of chemo, he would operate in December. By then, the mets should have shrunk to a point where he would be able to do wedge resections (the removal of a wedge-shaped section of lung tissue) rather than removing larger parts of my lung.

So it was back to the oncologist, Dr T, for me. My hair had just grown back, and once again I wasn't keen to lose it, which ruled out irinotecan. I also couldn't hack having the chemo pump again—because the beeping noise was so triggering it sent my body into shock—which tightened the list of options again. Lastly, I needed to have some form of quality of life, so we crossed off the most aggressive chemo that would make me cripplingly unwell.

I know I might sound demanding, but I know my limits. I know my body and I know what I need to stay motivated. My situation wasn't a simple case. If I knew I could do twelve months of aggressive treatment and be done with it, I would obviously have done that. But my cancer isn't curable—yet. It's not something I can overcome; it's something I have to live with.

This is my reality. For the rest of time, I will live in twelve-week blocks. I need to know I can survive one block to get to the next, and I need to live my life at the same time. Otherwise, what's the point?

After narrowing down the options, Dr T settled on Capecitabine, an oral chemo that is essentially the same drug as what I used to have in the pump, only I'd pop a few highly toxic tablets morning and night in exchange for the trauma-inducing beeping of the pump. Choose your fight, right? Originally, he had been hesitant to go down that road because the tablets are self-administered at home, and he knew I would stop taking

A non-ideal world

them if I had side effects. He wasn't wrong. As I learned the first time I had oral chemo, there's nothing you feel like doing less when you're sick than swallowing tablets that will make you sicker. But it was the only option that wouldn't make me lose my hair or go into trauma-induced shock.

The treatment plan involved taking 1500 milligrams of chemo in tablet form morning and night for two weeks, then having one week off. Alongside the chemo, I would keep doing my holistic treatments, including the Oncotherm, hydro-oxygen therapy with electromagnetic pulses, and my supplements. Ideally, I would do a three-hour session of therapy every second day (almost the equivalent of a part-time job). But in reality, I could only manage it twice a week.

As always, everything happened at once. The day I started chemo was the day we started painting our house. We had decided to sell because we needed more space for the revolving door of support we required when I was in treatment. That night was also the annual movie night fundraiser for the Jodi Lee Foundation, which I had been heavily involved in organising with my podcast co-host, Sophie. I was popping chemo pills, packing to move, running a fundraiser and planning Sophia's third birthday party. It was all happening.

Mercifully, I handled the oral chemo quite well. Sure, I was lethargic and tired, but I didn't have diarrhoea or vomiting, which was a first. Hallelujah. It wasn't until the final night of my first fortnight of chemo that I hit a wall. I was quite unwell and I spiralled.

It wasn't the treatment I was struggling with; it was everything else I was doing at the same time: being a mother, a wife, a friend, a daughter, a sister, a podcaster and an ambassador. I was trying to save my life—and the lives of others by sharing my story—and to live my life while doing so. My staunch independence was coming back to bite me on the arse.

When you're as headstrong and independent as me, everyone around you thinks you're okay because that's what you tell them. So when you relapse for a second or third time, they often don't even check in and ask how you are; they just assume you're okay like you were the last few times. And if they do ask, you say you're okay and they believe you. It's nobody's fault but your own. You believe that protecting everyone you love is the easiest way to save them from being burdened further by your illness. Of course, I didn't ask for it, either, but it felt easier for me to pretend than to place more trauma on my loved ones.

I was overwhelmed by all the things I was juggling (like every busy mum, ever) and I became withdrawn. I retreated into my shell and lost my voice. I needed to ask for help, but I couldn't say the words out loud.

Instead, I repeated a knee-jerk script: *Yeah, I'm okay. I'll be fine. Can't complain. Nothing compared to last time. Done it before, I can do it again. It's tough but I'm way tougher.*

A non-ideal world

These responses were pure deflection. That's my default. I think, deep down, I was trying to convince myself: if I said I was okay, maybe the words would trick my mind into believing so. That I was fine, that it was easier than last time, and the time before that. In reality, the fact that I even had anything to compare it to was fucked.

If I had answered honestly when asked how I was, I would have said I was slowly breaking. I would have explained how I'd spent more days furious at the world and at this horrific disease than ever before. I would have said that it doesn't get easier. Exposure therapy is bullshit—in fact, it gets a hell of a lot harder each time. The constant reminders, the frequency of the recurrence, the never-ending rotation that I seem to be stuck on: like the last minute of the washing machine cycle, it feels like it's never going to end.

I was a full 'yes man' for two years straight after diagnosis. In the latter half of 2024, though, I became a hermit. I claimed that I was saving all my extra energy for my family, but that was a lie. I was protecting my energy by avoiding anything that seemed even mildly uncontrollable. I figured, if I kept to myself, I wouldn't be reminded of what I was missing out on.

I struggled with navigating the relationships in my life. I felt like I was letting everyone down. When I had to cancel plans with friends, I was worried they would think I was a shit mate—after all, it seemed I could host a movie night or go to an event, but I couldn't go to dinner. I didn't want anyone to think I was using chemo as a cop-out. The truth was: going to brand events was part of my job, which was how I earned money, which was how I supported my daughter and paid for my expensive medical treatments. It mightn't have looked like work on Instagram, but it was part of the gig.

It was a classic catch 22. I needed money to pay for treatments to be well, but I needed to be well to make the money to pay for the treatments.

In an ideal world, I would be able to focus purely on my health and my daughter, but, newsflash: this isn't an ideal world.

I didn't know if I'd ever get calm seas in the storm that was my life, so I needed to learn to go with the flow. To keep my head above water, to float, to avoid drowning. It was hard when I so desperately wanted to be treated like myself—I loved that people saw me as more than my disease, more than a cancer patient. But I also needed people to remember that each day I was fighting for my life. How would I remind people without telling them? I'm yet to work this out.

I had to try to learn how to take a step back. I wanted to be active and involved in all the things. I wanted to be at kindy drop-off, at the footy, at the PR event and at the friend's baby shower. I wanted to be able to cook and clean for my family, to go to work and make a living, to show up and be a person. But sometimes it wasn't possible to do it all, to be it all. While I was taking chemo, I needed time to rest and to do my health sessions.

If I was out and about one day, I would often need a complete rest day afterwards. The exhaustion was real. Not even the people in my own house could recognise the level of my fatigue, because I'd become so good at hiding it from everyone. I managed to show up in the most basic ways just to get by. It was a really tough time to navigate.

I knew I wasn't alone in this predicament. Women so often feel the pressure to be everything to everyone. We're expected to work like we don't have kids and parent like we don't have a job. Add terminal cancer to the mix and the juggle becomes even more real. Motherhood, eh?

～

It was raining the week of Sophia's third birthday, but the sun came out to shine for her on the day of her party. It was a Sunday, the day before her actual birthday. We booked a winery just outside of Adelaide with a nice pinot for the adults and a big grassy lawn for the kids. Sophia had a *Frozen* cake, candles to blow out and lots of friends to ride the sugar rush with. It was such a chilled-out, beautiful day.

The day after—on her actual birthday—Sophia went to her first day of kindy. In South Australia, preschool and kindy are the same thing, and Aboriginal kids can enrol from the age of three. Soph was excited to start, but a little nervous because she didn't know all the kids' names yet, like she did at daycare.

Milestone moments such as Sophia's birthday and her first day at kindy are so precious to me. She is my purpose, my pride and joy.

My love for Sophia is like nothing I've ever known. I love Jeremy—he is the love of my life—but the love you feel for a child is different. It's not *more* than romantic love, just different. Both are all-consuming. Sometimes, when I look at Jeremy, I can feel my heart beating in my chest. There are moments when I look at Sophia and feel sure my heart will burst. And when I see them together? My heart is full.

I was watching Sophia ride her bike—at three!—when a realisation hit me: Soph had inherited my independence. She was fearless and confident and determined. Jeremy had been teaching Soph how to ride her bike, holding onto the handlebars as she pedalled. I was expecting to do the same when I took her out for a ride, but she sped off all on her own, a little BMX bandit. 'You can't catch me, I'm faster than you,' she yelled at me over her shoulder, leaving me in her dust.

'When did you turn into a teenager?' I asked.

Sophia is such a force of a child. I am complimented on her aura almost daily. Anyone who is lucky enough to meet our little girl tells me how special she is. It is the best thing to hear someone say that we've done an outstanding

A non-ideal world

job in the first three years of her life, especially considering all we were up against. Even as an only child, Soph isn't shy around other people and knows how to share (most of the time). She reminds me and Jeremy often that one day she will have a baby sibling—we just need to wait for the oven to cook them really well. See? She is ridiculously switched on.

Not long after Soph started kindy, her teacher told us, 'She'll be running this place soon.' She might have been one of the youngest kids, but she is mature beyond her years. Sometimes I wonder if Soph is purposely trying to grow up fast so I can see as much of her as possible. I wonder if she is so independent because she wants to put my mind at ease, to let me know she is going to be okay when I am gone. She is her mother's daughter, after all.

I've noticed Jeremy has started taking more photos and videos than he used to. I used to have to plead with him to take a selfie with me; now I catch him filming me and Soph on the couch or cooking dinner. They are candid videos capturing simple, everyday moments. We don't pose, we just are. I know he is taking them to show Sophia when she is older.

Cancer has taken a lot from me: my health, my time, my hair, my fertility. I expected those losses, but I didn't expect how much I would gain. I have a new perspective on life, motivation to share my story and spread awareness about bowel cancer, a new community, a stronger sense of self and greater empathy.

Cancer has also given me a new career path. It feels incredible to be able to earn a living from sharing my story, speaking at events and partnering with like-minded brands. When I do a keynote speech, I can see the effect my words have on people. Grown men well up with tears. People who have been touched by cancer are overcome with emotion, and everyone walks away with a newfound understanding: life is short, and precious, and it should be cherished.

Watching that realisation dawn on people reminds me of being back in the classroom. I feel the same satisfaction as I did when I saw a kid 'get it' in one of my lessons. Even though I was no longer a teacher at school, I was still teaching. And I hope I get to do it in a classroom again someday.

~

Once we got the green light from our lawyers and counsellors, it was full steam ahead on the surrogacy train. We ordered a home insemination kit off Amazon. We started tracking R's cycle and her basal body temperature, and ordered ovulation strips to know precisely when she was ovulating. R was keen for the process to be as 'natural' as possible—she's a bit scared of hospitals (same, girl, same)—so we decided to do the insemination at home. Hence the Amazon-delivered insemination kit. I was fascinated by how it all worked and what was involved.

Following R's cycle, we did the first insemination in July 2024. We had to get the timing just right. For the best chances, insemination has to happen during the fertile window, which is within six hours either side of ovulation.

When it was go time, Jeremy played his role. Basically, he had to ejaculate into a special cup. It was almost like a hospital urine sample jar, but with a rounded bottom to make it easier to get all the sperm out. It was also Jeremy's job to transfer the sperm from the cup into the syringe, at R's request (because I was pedantic about the speed in which it was done, and she didn't want to do it wrong).

My role in the process was supervisor, support person and hype girl. I was head researcher and chief operations officer. All of those titles were superficial, of course. I struggled not being able to contribute more actively. It was all up to Jeremy, R and the universe.

It wasn't a situation I ever imagined being in—standing in the kitchen with a woman from my home town, my husband and a syringe full of his sperm. Somehow, though, R made it feel entirely normal and easy. There was no awkwardness with her. R and Jeremy had a sibling-like friendship: she would take the piss out of him, and he would cop it on the chin. I liked that they had a bond, and it wasn't just me and R driving the whole thing. In a relatively short amount of time, we'd all become close. It's such an intimate thing to do—to create life together—that it was inevitable.

On the day I started chemo, when we began painting our house in anticipation for it going on the market, R came over and painted the back door for us. That's not a euphemism: she literally painted the back door. She slotted into our lives and family as though she was always meant to be there.

Back to business: once he'd filled the syringe, Jeremy passed the baton over to R. The syringe had a rounded tip, a bit like a tampon, for easy insertion, and there was an accompanying lubricant to help the swimmers get where they needed to go. R also needed to orgasm, to soften the cervix. Naturally, I bought her a cute little vibrator as a part of our insemination kit. It was all very high tech.

We left R to it and gave her some privacy. After inseminating the sperm, R had to keep the syringe inserted with her hips elevated for fifteen minutes. Then she put in a silicone menstrual cup to make sure nothing dripped out overnight.

After that, we waited. And waited. It's recommended to wait ten to twelve days after insemination before taking a pregnancy test. During that time, I found it hard to concentrate on anything else. It was all the more difficult not being able to talk about it. Jeremy and I decided not to tell anyone about our surrogacy attempt—not even my mum, or Zac (ha!). We didn't want any added pressure or to get other people's hopes up.

I messaged R to see if she had any (very) early symptoms. 'Does eating a whole packet of Tim Tams count?' she replied.

I immediately started craving a Tim Tam, and wondered if I was having sympathy symptoms.

When we mapped out the timeline, based on the date of insemination, we found out the baby would be due on our wedding anniversary. How poetic. It felt like it was too good to be true.

Ultimately, it was. R did a pregnancy test as soon as she was able to, and it came back positive. Sadly, it was a false positive. R wasn't pregnant. Our first insemination hadn't worked.

It was so painful. Even though we all knew that it's common not to fall pregnant the first time around, that knowledge didn't make it hurt any less. I was gutted. I felt deeply for everyone else who struggles with fertility issues, too. In that moment, I didn't know how I would buck up and do it all again the next month. I understood why people give up. It's such a roller-coaster ride of hope, worry, excitement and disappointment. I didn't know how long I could manage it for.

A month after our first attempt, we went through all the motions again—except this time, we had an added issue related to Jeremy's spleen. He had been in a collision during a game against the Gold Coast Suns, and started to feel pain in his sternum. The pain got worse after the game, and tests showed a small laceration to his spleen. He didn't need surgery, but he did need to rest and keep his heart rate stable. If Jeremy's heart rate lifted too high—say, from masturbating into a cup—he could bleed out and die.

It wasn't great timing. Obviously, I was worried about Jeremy, but I was also frustrated because I so desperately wanted the insemination to work, and timing was crucial. It was tough not having any control over the situation.

The circumstances for our second insemination attempt—that is, the inseminator being in hospital with a lacerated spleen—weren't ideal. We didn't like our chances, and we tried not to get ahead of ourselves. Even so, it was still a blow when R's pregnancy test came back negative.

It wasn't our time. All we could do was wait 28 days and pray for round three. Or four, or five. In 2024 I set the intention of being more patient, and the year put me to the test.

15

Remember me

The curtain was drawn, but I could still hear the lady next to me in the chemo suite chatting away. It was my second round of intravenous chemo—the one I had via the port in my chest—back in 2023, and I was having my bloods drawn by a nurse. Both her and I were listening in to the conversation happening on the other side of the curtain.

'There's this young lady married to a footballer in the paper, doing God's work, trying to spread awareness and being the spokesperson for bowel cancer,' the woman explained.

My nurse gave me a little grin and nodded at the curtain as if to say, 'Can I open it?'

'She's really young and has a sweet little girl. It's so sad,' the woman continued.

When the nurse opened the curtain, I looked over to her and smiled. 'That's me.'

'No, no,' she said. 'This girl has a toddler. She's married to a footballer.' She didn't recognise me. Admittedly I looked very, very different to my photo in the paper: my lush blonde locks were gone, and I was bald.

'Yeah, we're not married just yet, but you're talking about me,' I assured her. 'My daughter is Sophia, and I'm Kellie.'

A look of pride spread over her face. She swelled with it. She was excited to have met someone she'd been boasting about, someone she was inspired by and likely thought she'd never cross paths with. Pride was closely followed by a whole lot of pain and empathy. Her face crumpled with it; she knew the bleakness of what was to come. 'You're a warrior, my dear. You're going to change this world,' the woman told me. 'Your daughter is going to know you did it, too.'

I hoped the woman was right.

It wasn't a place I liked to dwell in—the time after I'd be gone—but it was somewhere I would visit. Of course, I'd thought about what would happen when I died. I wasn't scared for myself; I was scared for everyone I'd leave behind. I was scared for Jeremy, who would be a single parent. I was scared for Sophia, who would lose her mum. I was scared for my parents, who would have to bury their daughter.

I'd seen teddy bears with built-in voice recordings, and thought about getting one for Sophia so she could still hear my voice. I'd written letters in my head for her 18th and 21st birthdays, her last day of school and her wedding. I hadn't actually written the words on paper, though. Doing that would make it real, make it inevitable, make me admit defeat.

I believed that the moment I gave in to the idea of not being here, the disease would overcome me. I wasn't ready for that moment. Until I ran out of options and second opinions—and until I was explicitly told I was at the end of the road—I was going to keep on keeping on. It was all I knew how to do.

We had the same approach to our surrogacy. When R's period arrived two days early after our third insemination attempt, we were crushed. I tried not to let my disappointment show, especially to R. I didn't want her to feel that she had somehow failed. It doesn't work like that. There was nothing she could have done or not done to make the insemination stick. It was just the way it went.

Still, the failed cycles felt like heavy weights. Once again, something completely out of my control was having a negative impact on me. Is it any wonder I became a bit of a control freak?

In the lead-up to insemination attempt four, we did all the things. R booked in to have acupuncture (even though she's afraid of needles—such a trooper) and her naturopath prescribed her progesterone to help prepare her uterus lining.

R flew to Adelaide from the Eyre Peninsula, where she was based. We'd experienced delayed flight after delayed flight, acupuncture appointments cancelled, hope running out.

There Must Be More

We'd tracked R's cycle so closely for four months, and on our fourth try her hormones decided to peak two days earlier than expected. Because of that, we missed the 30–40 per cent chance of pregnancy window, and had just a 10–15 per cent chance by the time she landed. Once an egg is ovulated, it only survives 12–24 hours before being reabsorbed.

The time was ticking. Our chances were becoming slim. I was trying to distract myself with other success stories, but I couldn't stop watching the clock. The window was so tight, and I couldn't bear the thought of having to wait another month for it to open again.

Surrogacy is hard. Trying to conceive naturally is difficult enough, but adding into the mix an eight-hour drive between us and our surrogate, and the fact our three lives didn't just stop to allow us to make a baby, navigating the process was so much trickier than expected. Both myself and R fell pregnant 'easily' with our firsts. So we assumed, naively, that we would have a similar experience now. At only 28, R was in her peak, after all. But it was starting to look a lot less likely.

I was craving a newborn. I so desperately wanted to give Sophia a sibling. I wanted nothing more than to actually get to enjoy the first year of motherhood, to rewrite the narrative. But I started to wonder, at what cost? Not just financially—as you can imagine, the process had taken a toll on our bank account—but emotionally. The constant heartache each month when another cycle didn't work, when we got that negative test result, when we realised we may have missed ovulation altogether—it was another very constant reminder that my body had been through hell, that my body had failed me. That my life wasn't what I'd expected or hoped for. That Sophia might be an only child.

I didn't want to accept any of that. But how was I supposed to look after myself, and make sure I was getting back to my best health, if all I could focus on was the loss each month? My heart couldn't take it. My body didn't need the stress. How was I supposed to get through it? How could I control the uncontrollable?

They weren't even questions I could ask my loved ones, because we'd chosen not to speak about the surrogacy until we had something concrete to say. Only a couple of friends knew what we were going through. Those friends checked in with me, but not too often, in case it triggered something, which I appreciated.

On top of everything, Jeremy's spleen injury sidelined him for the remainder of the season—a season in which his team made it to the preliminary finals. Understandably, that was tough on him. I was conscious of Jeremy's emotions and didn't want to add to the load on his shoulders. He's lucky he has great shoulders, but still.

~

I hate funerals. I've only been to one funeral in my adult life because I hate them so much. The funeral I went to was for my brother's godparent's dad, who was also the grandpa of one of my best friends from school. We were close family friends—so much so, I considered my friend my cousin. I come from a small town, remember? I went to the funeral to support the family. I didn't have it in me to last too long at the wake, though.

There's a running joke in my family that I'll do anything to get out of a funeral. When my uncle Paul died, and I had to break the news to his daughter, I couldn't go to his funeral because I was on a flight to Bali. I put the photos together for the funeral slideshow, but I couldn't be there on the day.

Likewise, I was on a flight to Norway when my grandmother died. My grandma had paid for the flight—she was so excited for me to experience my grandpa's homeland—so I knew she wouldn't have wanted me to turn straight around and fly all the way back to Australia.

Of course, I would have liked to be there for my family and to pay my respects, but I wasn't sad to miss the morbid formalities.

It's written in my will that when I die, there's not to be a funeral. No. I don't want one. They're horrible and sad and expensive. I don't want people standing around ugly crying in public. Cry at home, and then go to the pub and have a beer in my honour instead!

'But what if I want to give you a funeral?' Jeremy has asked me.

'Well, do it in your bedroom, on your own,' I said.

It was a flippant comment from Jeremy. I didn't think he would actually want to have a funeral for me—he would never go against my wishes—but he also doesn't have the same aversion to funerals as I do. In mid-2024 he travelled to Melbourne for the funeral of his aunt's ex-husband, whom he hadn't seen in years.

Funerals are the *done* thing. But I'd never stuck to the traditional path, so why would I start?

Instead of a funeral, I liked the idea of having my ashes spread over the ocean. Don't stand around a casket in a funeral parlour. Take an esky to the beach and sink your toes in the sand. Don't dwell on the loss, celebrate the life.

~

Since I began sharing my story, became a Jodi Lee Foundation ambassador and started the *Sh!t Talkers* podcast, I'd received messages from people across the country. Some were from relatives of people with cancer thanking me for sharing my lived experiences; others were from recently diagnosed patients at the start of their journey; and some were from young girls who'd booked in to see a doctor after dismissing their tummy troubles as a gluten intolerance or IBS for too long.

There Must Be More

Often the feedback was second-hand, from friends or friends of friends, who relayed conversations to me. When I overheard the woman in the chemo suite while I was having my bloods drawn, it was one of the first times I felt like what I was doing was working and worth it. As bizarre as it was, hearing a stranger tell my story was so cool—I could see how far my message had spread.

One day Jeremy went to get a tattoo and the artist was talking about me! The guy needling ink into my husband's shin had heard my story and knew my face.

I'd heard Jezz telling others how proud he was of me and my advocacy work, too. 'Even on her shit days she doesn't sit in the corner and sook,' he said. 'She just keeps rocking up. She's the best mum to Sophia, and the best wife to me. She cooks us beautiful dinners, despite whatever she's going through. She's so strong, I love that about Kell.'

When I posted on social media asking if anyone had a lead on a Taylor Swift ticket for sale, one of my followers slid into my DMs. She very generously offered for me to join her and her daughter in the A Reserve section at the show. She explained that she'd only recently—weeks earlier—started following me, after a friend told her my story. That friend had been experiencing unusual symptoms and had gone to see a doctor because of my advocacy.

Karma might be Taylor's boyfriend, but it's also a spare ticket to a sold-out show.

Of course, I didn't become an advocate for the stadium seats. I'd been public with my experiences in the hope of helping others. And that hope had come true.

I wanted people to know that cancer doesn't discriminate. It doesn't matter if you're young, old, rich, poor, fit or not: cancer could impact any one of us. It doesn't care if you're a new mum. It couldn't give a fuck if you're the healthiest and happiest you've ever been. I hoped my efforts would be recognised and responded to; that those who'd met me would be more aware of their own beings; that those who were touched by my story would be impacted in whatever way they needed: whether it gave them a push in the right direction, the confidence to seek help in any capacity, or even a reminder that no one ever knows anyone's whole story.

In saying that, a diagnosis isn't a death sentence. People can survive cancer, and also thrive in spite of it (like me). Advancements are being made every day and survival rates are improving alongside them. Cancer isn't one-size-fits-all. The symptoms and treatments differ from case to case. One thing that is the same across the board, though, is the importance of early detection. The sooner cancer is found, the better.

That's why I am so damn passionate about encouraging people to trust their guts. To get checked out. To advocate for themselves. To listen to their bodies. To prioritise their health.

There Must Be More

In the last couple of years, I've been getting requests to do keynote speeches and be on university panels about cancer. At first, I didn't know what I had to add to these important conversations. I'm not a doctor! And I'm not yet a cancer survivor. What do I know? It turns out, quite a lot.

So many cancer stories are told by people who've overcome the disease, or by the people who've been left behind. The message is usually 'I beat cancer' or 'In loving memory of'. It's rare to hear from someone actively living with a terminal illness (probably because they're just trying to get through each day in the trenches—I get it). That's where I come in. I feel a sense of responsibility to use my voice, to share my experiences and to talk about uncomfortable shit. Figuratively and literally.

I'm not a fan of the B-word: brave. When I am called brave—for living with cancer—I feel uncomfortable. I don't consider myself to be brave for the way I live my life, because I have no choice in the matter. If I don't live, I will die. That isn't an option for me. I don't think that has made me brave, it's just made me stubborn.

What I do think is brave is being vulnerable. It hasn't been easy stepping into the spotlight and opening myself up to judgement and criticism. It hasn't been easy talking about the deepest, darkest moments of my life. It hasn't been easy reliving my trauma and putting it on display.

But good things don't come easily. We all know that.

And something good has to come out of it all. It simply *has* to.

~

Six months on from starting that fresh round of chemo, not much has changed on the treatment front. Chemo continues to be part of my reality. I didn't end up having surgery in December 2024 as I had hoped—quelle surprise—but it's on my wishful-thinking bingo card for 2025.

Right bang in the middle of that bingo card is our hope to also grow our family. I would have loved to share an update on our surrogacy journey, but, sadly, there isn't one to share yet.

Despite all the continued challenges and uncertainty, one thing is for sure: life is still worth living.

The thing that has changed recently is my headspace. I feel like I'm leaving my hermit era and entering a new phase—coming out of my shell, if you will. When life feels overwhelming, I like to remind myself that there was a time when the busiest I could be was rolling from one side of the bed to the other. I'm now focusing on making the most of all of the incredible opportunities being thrown my way and sharing my voice as loud as I can while I have it.

~

There Must Be More

It's strange to think about how you'll be remembered. It's not a question many twenty-somethings have to ponder. And yet, here I am, thinking about it.

I don't want to be remembered for having cancer; I want to be remembered for the way I responded to having cancer. I didn't choose cancer—no one does—but I do choose life. I choose not just to survive but to thrive. I wake up every day and refuse to give up. I do it in spite of my diagnosis. I do it regardless of my prognosis. I do it for my daughter.

Of course, I want to stick around for my husband, parents and friends, too, but my intense desire to be there for Sophia is something else entirely. It is an overwhelming sense of protection for my child. Everyone else in my life is old enough to know what is going on and to work out a way to cope without me, but Sophia isn't. She's too young to picture a life without her mum, and it is my mission every single day to ensure she doesn't have to.

One day, Sophia will know what I went through to be there for her milestones—turning three, starting kindy, learning to ride a bike—and I hope there will be comfort in that knowledge.

I hope to be remembered not just for the unfair battle I faced, but for the courage with which I navigated it, and the lives I touched along the way. I want to be associated with empowerment and strength, not grief and loss. I want to live on through my advocacy, and through the way I've tried to highlight the reality of what everyday people living with invisible disabilities go through. I aspire to be the lightbulb moment, the change in the campaign for awareness.

Most importantly I want to be remembered as the world's most loving mother, who faced immense challenges with grace and determination. For Sophia, my greatest legacy is the love and resilience I've tried to model for her. I want her, above everyone, to remember that even in the darkest days there is always light to be found and strength to be drawn from.

When people google 'Kellie Finlayson' I hope it will read: 'A mother, wife, daughter, sister and best friend. Kellie Finlayson was a colorectal cancer thriver. Despite the shadow of illness, she illuminated the path for others to find their own strength and voice.'

When people remember me, I hope they'll be reminded to choose kindness in every breath.

In the end, if my journey has inspired even one person to seek help sooner, to speak more openly or to face their own struggles with a bit more courage, then my story has been worth telling. I want my life and work to serve as a beacon of hope and a call to action for others.

When I stood opposite Jeremy at the altar in 2023, I promised to be his best friend for as long as I was able to, to be the best mum to Sophia in the time I had with her, and to continue to guide her even after I was gone. 'I hope I can keep making you, Soph and our family and friends proud,' I said to my husband, who I knew would one day be my widower.

The sentiment still stands. And somehow, against all odds, I'm still standing, too.

Acknowledgements

Kellie
Bringing this memoir to life has been a deeply personal and transformative journey, and I am profoundly grateful to everyone who walked alongside me during this process.

Alley, when I grow up, I want to be just like you. Truly, you are one of a kind.

Sharing such vulnerable moments from my life hasn't always been easy, but knowing how many lives I'm impacting—and even saving—makes it all so worth it. The grace and courage I've found along the way are reflections of the incredible people surrounding me.

To my daughter, Sophia: You'll never know just how much you saved me, but I'll spend the rest of my life reminding you how proud I am to be your mum and how deeply I love you.

To my husband, Jeremy: You will always be my person. We've faced what could have broken us, yet we've come through stronger. Thank you for letting me share so many 'behind-the-scenes' moments, knowing that everything I do is for the greater good.

To my family, especially my mum: You are not only my rock, but also Jeremy's and Sophia's. We are so lucky to have you. To my dad, thank you for holding the fort while Mum held all of us. And to my brother, Jake: I'll never forget how much you love me—you remind everyone (with a few tears) every time you've had a sip of alcohol!

To my friends: You know who you are. To those who have been there every step of the way, showing up in every way I could ever need, I'm endlessly grateful. To my bridesmaids, my soul sisters, my comforts—thank you for everything.

To the team at Allen & Unwin: Thank you for believing in me more than I ever believed in myself. You've given me the gift of becoming a published author and bringing this important book into the world. I cannot thank you enough.

And finally, to my readers (OMG, pinch me!): Thank you for coming along on this wild journey. I love you all.

Alley

I was in a sauna with my friend Mia when she told me about this podcast she'd listened to, which made her book in to see a doctor. 'This girl was 25 and thought she had a gluten

Acknowledgements

intolerance because that was all the rage at the time, but it was bowel cancer,' Mia explained. The girl was Kellie. And the very next week, Kellie messaged me on Instagram about her book.

I've seen first-hand the power of Kellie's story, and I feel honoured to have helped tell that story in this book. Kell is one of a kind, a force of nature and bright spark in the world. I want to thank her for being so candid, dedicated and raw during this process, and for so generously sharing the reality of life with a terminal illness.

I also want to thank Jeremy, Jane, Jess, Kobi, Christina, Brya, Tina and everyone else who provided their insights and support for the book.

I'm enormously thankful to our brilliant publisher Sally Heath, project editor Courtney Lick, copyeditor Brooke Lyons, OG visionary Tessa Feggans and the entire team at Allen and Unwin for all their faith and magic.

Personally, I need to thank my loved ones—Mum, Sophie, Thor, Malili, Meg, Ilma and Mia—for holding me upright on the hard days. Daisy and Fae for being my emotional support animals, and James for being my biggest fan. Thank you, truly.

Kellie Finlayson and Jodi Lee Bowel Cancer Foundation

A special partnership

The Jodi Lee Bowel Cancer Foundation has had the privilege of standing alongside Kellie Finlayson while she has courageously shared her story with the world. As a dedicated Jodi Lee Bowel Cancer Foundation ambassador since April 2023 and the face of our *Trust Your Gut* campaign, Kellie has been instrumental in raising awareness about bowel cancer—its symptoms and the importance of acting early. In her words, 'Bowel cancer doesn't discriminate, bowel cancer doesn't know or care how old you are. So YOU have to care, and YOU have to trust your gut.'

Kellie is a prominent force in advocating for your health and trusting your gut when something doesn't feel right. Her heartfelt story resonates with so many, offering hope, strength and insights.

Her journey continues to inspire all who hear it, and it's because of her that we truly believe in the transformative power of storytelling.

About the Jodi Lee Bowel Cancer Foundation

The Jodi Lee Bowel Cancer Foundation empowers people to take active steps to prevent bowel cancer and live healthy lives. Each year, the Jodi Lee Bowel Cancer Foundation reaches millions of Australians through its national initiatives to fight bowel cancer—one bowel screening test at a time, one awareness campaign at a time, one story at a time.

Jodi's story

In 2008, Jodi and her husband Nick were living in Vietnam, where Nick was working. Happily together for 12 years, they were having the time of their lives with their two young children.

Nick was away when Jodi rang him complaining of constipation, abdominal pain and some bloating. Her doctor quickly recognised an obstruction in her bowel and ordered scans. Jodi had cancer and the tumour had all but blocked her bowel. She was only 39 years old.

After emergency surgery to remove the cancer, Jodi and Nick received the worst news possible: the cancer had spread to Jodi's lymph nodes and liver. At best, she only had two years to live.

One of the hardest things Jodi and Nick had to do was tell their children, Jack and Arabella, that their mum was going to die. Jodi passed away on 16 January 2010, a few days before her 42nd birthday.

Before Jodi's diagnosis, she was fit and healthy. She had no family history of bowel cancer and no symptoms whatsoever, which is typical of bowel cancer. The saddest part of Jodi's story is that it could have had a different ending if her bowel cancer had been detected early.

With that simple fact as the driving force, the Jodi Lee Bowel Cancer Foundation was established in 2010.

The Jodi Lee Bowel Cancer Foundation is a leading voice for the prevention and early detection of bowel cancer. Each year, the Foundation reaches millions of Australians, arming them with the knowledge they need to prevent bowel cancer and the motivation to be proactive about their health.

Jodi was a radiant woman—full of warmth and kindness. Though her time with us was far too short, her light continues to shine brightly through every life saved.

Bowel cancer
The facts
- Bowel cancer is the leading cancer killer in 25–44-year-old Australians.
- Incidences of bowel cancer in people under 50 have increased 266% in the last thirty years.
- Bowel cancer is the second most common cause of cancer-related death in Australia.
- Australia has one of the highest rates of bowel cancer in the world.

- Each year over 15,500 people are diagnosed with bowel cancer in Australia.
- Bowel cancer claims over 5,300 lives in Australia every year.
- Acting quickly when you first notice symptoms is the key, because if detected early, over 90% of bowel cancer cases can be successfully treated.
- Regular bowel screening—which looks for traces of blood in your poo—is one of the most effective ways to detect bowel cancer early.

The symptoms

Regardless of your age, speak to your GP immediately if you experience any of the following symptoms:
- Blood in your poo, even if only occasional
- A change in bowel habits for longer than two weeks, such as:
    - Going to the toilet more frequently
    - Constipation
    - Loose or watery bowel movements
    - Feeling that the bowel does not completely empty
    - Bowel movements that are narrower than usual
- Frequent gas pains, bloating, fullness or cramps
- Persistent and severe abdominal pain
- A lump in your stomach or rectum
- Unexplained feelings of tiredness, breathlessness or a lack of energy
- Unexplained weight loss or vomiting.

Kellie Finlayson and Jodi Lee Bowel Cancer Foundation

Free symptom checker

The Jodi Lee Bowel Cancer Foundation Symptom Checker guides you through a series of questions, while providing helpful advice and information based on the user answers provided. If the Symptom Checker recommends you make an appointment with a GP, we urge you to prioritise booking that appointment—it might just save your life.

The Symptom Checker tool is available to use for free: www.trustyourgut.com.au

Bowel screening test

The simple at-home screening test looks for blood in your poo—a common sign of bowel abnormality—that might be invisible to the naked eye. It is not a test for cancer.

If you are between the ages of 50 to 74, you will receive a free bowel screening test kit in the mail every two years, thanks to the Australian Government's National Bowel Cancer Screening Program (NBCSP).

If you are between the ages of 45 to 49, you can now opt in to receive this free home bowel screening test kit from the Australian Government. You can join the National Bowel Cancer Screening Program by requesting your first bowel screening kit at www.ncsr.gov.au/boweltest or by calling the National Cancer Screening Register (NCSR) Contact Centre on 1800 627 701.

If you aren't eligible for a free kit, you can purchase a bowel screening test from the Jodi Lee Foundation website: https:/jodileefoundation.org.au/bowel-screening

Only 44 per cent of Australians aged 50–74 complete their free bowel screening test when it arrives in the mail from the Australian Government, but if bowel cancer is detected early, we can treat over 90 per cent of bowel cancer cases. If we can increase participation in the National Bowel Cancer Screening Program to 60 per cent by 2040, we will save an additional 84,000 lives. If you have lost or misplaced your test, request a replacement by contacting the National Bowel Cancer Screening Program at www.ncsr.gov.au/boweltest or 1800 627 701.

Remember: early detection saves lives.